GITA *for* JACOB

A book about a book
Come, discover this timeless treasure

NAFISA J. APTEKAR

Gita for Jacob
Copyright © 2024 by Nafisa J. Aptekar

All rights reserved. No part of this publication may be reproduced, distributed, or transmitted in any form or by any means, including photocopying, recording, or other electronic or mechanical methods, without the prior written permission of the author, except in the case of brief quotations embodied in critical reviews and certain other non-commercial uses permitted by copyright law.

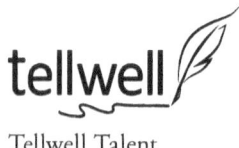

Tellwell Talent
www.tellwell.ca

ISBN
978-1-77962-152-8 (Hardcover)
978-1-77962-151-1 (Paperback)
978-1-77962-153-5 (eBook)

DEDICATION

This book is dedicated to Jacob and to you, the reader

TABLE OF CONTENTS

Preface vii
Introduction ix

Chapter

1: Wrong Thinking Is A Big Problem In Life 1
2: Right Knowledge Is A Solution To Our Problems 5
3: Becoming Eligible To Search The Right Knowledge
   Step 1: Karm Yoga.. 9
4: Becoming Eligible To Search The Right Knowledge
   Step 2: Daily Sadhana 17
5: Progressing To The Next Step: The Concept Of Seva 20
6: Continuing The Right Steps With The
   Right Attitude: Vivek, Bhava, Sankalpa. Shraddha,
   Sharangati, Dharma..24
7: The Right Attitude Needs A Clean Container:
   The Three Gunas 30
8: Making The Container Dazzle: Tapas...............................45
9: The Law Of Karma..63

Appendix 1: Before You Start The Actual Study Of The
             Bhagavad Gita..79
Appendix 2: Meanings Of Words In Bold And More............. 81
Appendix 3: Books I Wish To Recommend 90
Appendix 4: Youtube Podcasts 92
About The Author..93

PREFACE

Jacob is my husband. He is Jewish. He is 71 years old and he has not yet ever picked up the Bhagavad Gita. Neither have our two adult sons. So, I have written a book about why one should study the **Bhagavad Gita As It Is by A.C Bhaktivedanta Swami Prabhupada.**

For those of you who have not heard about the Bhagavad Gita, it is a text from the ancient Indian scriptures, written as a set of questions and answers between Arjuna, a warrior prince and his teacher and friend Sri Krishna. In this conversation, Sri Krishna helps Arjuna overcome his inner conflict so that he can perform the right action.

The subject matter may seem alien to you, as it seemed to me a decade and half earlier. However, when you study, assimilate, and apply the knowledge the Bhagavad Gita provides, you have a user manual for life. The Bhagavad Gita was written five thousand years ago and has stood the test of time.

Book stores in malls and airports flaunt many self-help books prominently, books to help you discover the secret of happiness and books on stress management. Yet in these times of the mental health pandemic, I believe the Gita can offer a solution like no other.

I have written this book in the hope that it awakens your desire to try something you have never tried before and embark on the journey to seek further as I have done.

INTRODUCTION

Why is ***The Bhagavad-Gita*** so unique? Why term it a user manual for life?

Why is it different from the countless self-help books already published? Because it contains the real secret to find the happiness that you seek. This is true whether or not you follow a formal religion. Neither do you need to convert to Hinduism.

Yes, we spend much time, money, and effort seeking happiness and relief from stress. But even after reading many 'how to find happiness' books, enjoying expensive vacations, downing the finest whisky or smoking a zillion cigarettes, and if nothing else works, trying a Xanax, you may find that instead of bliss you are still a mess.

I am a physician, practicing family medicine in the community in Ontario, Canada. This system of diagnosis and treatment works well to cure diseases of the body like infection, tumors and high blood pressure, but where the mind is concerned, its reductionist approach does not do too well. Psychiatry, the specialty of mental health, lacks a definition of 'happiness'. The Bhagavad Gita does: The book says happiness is your true and natural state. Rediscovering this natural state is the secret to feeling good consistently. Happiness is **not** something we can create or buy.

This dearth of not finding happiness is creating the mental health pandemic we see all around. The T.V. talks about it, the magazines give statistics, the experts dole out grim predictions, but no one has the solution. According to the Mental Health Commission of Canada, in any given year, one in five Canadians experience mental illness. About 21.4% of the working population in Canada currently experience mental health problems that can affect their productivity and many Canadians miss work each week due to mental illness. In the clinic, I see factory employees come with headaches that make them miss work, families falling apart because of anger issues in one parent, students presenting with completed self questionnaires on attention deficit disorder, citing it as a reason they cannot focus on school.

The problem is huge but unfortunately, there are no simple how-to instructions for happiness. We are not IKEA furniture which one opens and does the assembly as per instructions. We are, so to speak, already assembled.

When the mind is more like a pot already filled with water, one cannot fill more water into it. In other words, when one is so used to a set of thoughts, one needs to remove the layers of conditioning.

Where does one start? Become eligible for the make over. Believe me or not, it begins with the food. If one fills one's body with junk, one becomes junk. Sri Krishna says do not eat mere food, eat **prasad**. He clearly instructs what can be eaten and what cannot be eaten in Chapter 17 of the Gita.

But hey! Don't jump to Chap 17. Don't be the analyser. Imperfect senses cannot understand perfect knowledge. When the door of wisdom opens, one begins to understand. But one has to make oneself eligible to receive the knowledge. Help is available. The Bhagavad Gita explains how to proceed on this path.

Then the daily practice must begin. Once you have understood how to declutter the mind, you have to learn how to put in place the knowledge. This implementation will need discipline. Without discipline and application, your knowledge will remain only theoretical. (*From Swami Muktananda: The Ranveer show 370*).

The reader needs to be open to concepts which may be new.

1. **Atma**: spirit/consciousness/self: The concept that we are spiritual beings having a human experience (embodied being). The word soul can be used but is not as accurate as the term atma.
2. **Karma:** action as in thought, speech and physical work: The embodied being cannot remain inactive except in deep sleep.
3. **Yog:** to join. Join what? Us to the one who created us,

References to the actual Bhagavad Gita have been noted numerically as B.G. Chapter number verse number for example B.G.2:22 for your easy reference.

Through this book, you will notice that I have strayed from the actual 'Bhagavad Gita as It Is' in different sections and gone into medicalese, patient stories and references to other books and resources to convey a point. These have also been a part of my journey which I want to share with you.

It is grace that brought the Gita into my life and hopefully the same blessing will shower upon you. If I could bring about a change in my life, so can you. The Gita does not use fear or greed to spark obeisance to the Supreme, the emotion is **bhava:** A mix of affection, devotion and love.

You cannot have **bhava** for someone/something you do not know. But when you enroll for Sri Krishna's tutorship, changes begin. If Prabhupad could make the hippies of New Jersey and California dance in ecstasy by chanting the mantra he taught them and give up intoxication and meat, change is possible for all of us who are motivated to challenge our attitudes.

Also holding this knowledge, you will not ask yourself what the future holds, because you will know who holds the future. *(from Chaitanya Charan Das https://www.youtube.com/ live/5yXntX6pe01?si=hA1TU7nMTuQmtjx3)*

CHAPTER 1

WRONG THINKING IS A BIG PROBLEM IN LIFE

What stresses you, Jacob?

One morning, one of your old University classmates sent you a message. He is inviting himself to our home for a few days and requires you to take him and his wife sightseeing in Toronto. Dates were specified, no requests were made.

At breakfast, you were irritable. We did not focus on the delicious flavor of the oatmeal.

Who does he think he is? Does he not have the courtesy to ask whether we are okay to host them or even to wait for an invite?

In the evening, the topic continued. We debated and came to a conclusion. Finally, we decided we did not want the unwanted guests.

A two second message took up at least an hour of mental space. Could you have minimised that time? Sixty minutes of happiness less in your life.

What if we had been able to deal with the unwanted classmate situation without the stress?

What if we had been able to view the problem differently and not let it stress us out?

The Bhagavad Gita begins with a description of a stressful situation. Prince Arjuna, the warrior prince is faced with two choices on the battlefield: to fight or not to fight. He chooses not to and puts down his weapon. He thinks that it is the right decision.

What is wrong thinking?

Wrong thinking is the thought process that prevents us from having the right perspective and leads to a faulty decision.

Arjuna was overwhelmed in his decision-making process. He had to fight a battle against his own family members to regain his kingdom. On one hand was his identity as a warrior and on the other as a member of his clan. Should he avoid killing his own family members or should he consider his duty as warrior first and fight to regain his kingdom? His decision to put down his weapon was the wrong decision because of wrong thinking and Sri Krishna had to step in to educate.

In the Bhagavad Gita, Sri Krishna says we have the wrong thought processes because of ***avidya*** (**ignorance**). It is what the knowledge of the Gita aims to remove.

In the present age, wrong thought processes coupled with societal influences are spearheading the devastating increase in the incidence of mental health problems. In the midst of affluence and the unprecedented technological developments of the 21st century, an increasing number of people are living lives of stunted awareness. When they are younger, the busyness of their lives, the constant yo-yo syndrome of so-called work life balance: (work/entertainment/work/vacation/work) offers some protection to some. The problems worsen as people progress to senior citizenship. Free medical care, old age security and Canada Pension Plan cannot stall it. My patients come and say "Old age sucks" But the fear of death keeps many wanting to remain alive. So, they retire to retirement homes, advance to assisted living and end up in nursing homes. You will be surprised at the number of nursing homes in Ontario. A new disease has even been coined seen only in the nursing homes: It is called Inappropriate Sexual Behaviour in long term care facilities with an incidence of 1.8 to 2.5% *(Canadian geriatrics society journal of CME)*. Twelve medications have been recommended for treatment including hormones to suppress the libido. But old age, once the ignorance is removed need not be the period of prolonged suffering that my patients describe it to be.

A wrong thought process also makes a problematic situation doubly stressful. Buddha tells the parable of the two arrows. He says suffering is like a man hit by two arrows. A man is hit by worldly situations, that is the first arrow: be it war, natural disasters, disease, financial or relationship problems. What is this second arrow? The second arrow is our reaction to the first. If you remove the second arrow, the first arrow would not sting as much alone.

Many people get overwhelmed by the first arrow that the world aims at them and are further destroyed by the reactionary arrow.

The story of Maya:

Maya worked as a chef in an office canteen since 2015. Her work revolved around cutting, chopping and prepping food. Her supervisor decided to fire the third member of the team and Maya ended up doing the work of two people. This was not kind on her right shoulder and in 2018 she developed a condition called bicipital tendinitis, which happens to people who overuse their shoulders at work and end up fraying the tendons in the shoulder joint. She also had to work close to a vent fan for about three to four hours a day. This impaired her hearing, and the Workers Compensation Board got involved. Maya got put off the work that she once loved, but was painful to do anymore, spiralled into a gloom of depression as the shoulder injury showed no sign of healing, the workers disability contribution stopped and money problems started.

Her psychiatrist started her on an antidepressant, then an antipsychotic to stabilize the symptoms. Fast forward to 2024, Maya continues to remain off work, she has developed mild diabetes and remains as sad and lost as ever. Her 15-year marriage has crumbled and I have now completed the paperwork to apply for the Canada Disability Pension Plan for her at the age of 45.

The story of Arun:

His downward slope started in 2017, though the seeds of the illness, of self doubt and poor self worth had been sown much earlier. Unfortunately, instead of seeking help, he self treated – with alcohol. He had been living away from his wife and children in another province for two years because of his job, had started drinking excessively and had stopped exercising completely. When he got to the stage of full-blown substance abuse disorder, he did come sporadically to ask for help with withdrawal symptoms but could not progress to even conventional allopathic treatment of his disease.

The withdrawal symptoms would be worse in the morning, Arun would have his first drink at noon and feel better. He expressed a desire to stop drinking, but the motivation always left him when face to face with the bottle. I suggested a medicine that would take alcohol cravings away and gave him a script. But it was too late. My last counselling session with Arun was in May 2022. The young 34-year-old hung himself in his garage two months later.

These stories are just two of many that did not need to have been written, if the main character could have been rescued.

CHAPTER 2

RIGHT KNOWLEDGE IS A SOLUTION TO OUR PROBLEMS

When Prince Arjuna was faced with his problem (in the **battle of Kurukshetra**) he started lamenting. and became despondent.

He sat down and said 'I will not fight' Overwhelmed with sorrow he said 'it is better to live by begging than kill my most noble teachers'.

He turned to Krishna for help: 'Now I am confused and have lost all composure. In this condition I am asking You to tell me for certain what is best for me. Please instruct me'

Krishna did not kick start a positive self talk series

In the dramatic space of a battlefield where many thousands fully trained, experienced professional soldiers had come with the intention to fight, Krishna suddenly orchestrated a pause for one hour and in that one hour, where the warriors were there, the battlefield was there, the weapons of war were there, but the warrior seemed to have lost his will for the war, Sri Krishna brought the Bhagavad Gita as the literature to help him to first win the internal conflict before he could be victorious in winning the external war. Today's society is so obsessed with winning the external battle (money, fame, success) before they can win the internal conflict, that the world today is experiencing 300 million cases of depression (*excerpted from Gaurang das Prabhu YouTube Podcast The Ranveer show 318*)

Yes, today the Gita is needed ever more than ever before.

Stanley (name changed) came to the clinic this morning, stating he had a problem with his blood pressure. Stanley is 33 years old. He mostly came with his young family for regular check ups and baby problems for his two little ones, hardly ever for himself, so the high blood pressure concern sounded an alarm

The true story peeked out. His wife and he had separated two weeks ago. This life shaking event drove him to marijuana and drove up his blood pressure. Marijuana for succor? Easily available in Canada. The bud shops are open in the malls even on a Sunday evening.

The saddest thought that grips me at such instances of unexpected human suffering is I perceive I have the dose of the right medicine in my hand, my patient is sitting there right in front of me, but I cannot administer it to him. I want to shout 'take it 'but my voice falls silent. I instead meekly hand him the script for the anti – anxiety pill.

I cannot talk to Stanley about the Gita, hopefully the temporary benzodiazepine will cause less damage than the marijuana. Will he heal? Will his young life be turned into a morass of cynicism just because his beautiful family fell apart?

Likely. Stanley, like thousands of others, does not know where to start.

Will he be able to listen and understand the real truth? As Prabhupada says in his purport (B.G.2:12): A common man with all the four defects of human fragility (imperfect senses, propensity for cheating, certainty of committing mistakes and certainty of being disillusioned) is unable to hear that which is worth hearing.

Are you ready to hear, Jacob? Or will you just close off this book and switch on the T.V? Too much heavy stuff you may say. I have other interesting things to occupy my mind.

Yes, it is heavy stuff for a mind already stuffed, the pot already brimming with water.

Coming back to Sri Krishna: He asks Arjuna. 'What are you lamenting for? Whom are you going to kill in the war?'

He throws a mind blower at Arjuna: 'You are lamenting that you will be slaying your uncles and teachers if you agree to fight, but neither are you the slayer nor they the ones who will be slain.'

So, who are you?

Sri Krishna introduces the concept that we are immortal and an immortal being cannot be killed. The real you is the consciousness that lights up the body and mind and is immortal. Yet this immortal aspect cannot be realized by us. We are licking the bottle of honey from outside. One cannot have a taste of the honey unless one opens the bottle.

It is imperative we know who we are now, before we fritter our entire lives feeding our bodies with food, sex and other pleasures, titillating our minds with different toys, completing our bucket lists until at the ripe old age of 80 or 90 when the eyes are finally dimmed or cataracted, the teeth are either implanted or dentured, the ears are likely equipped with hearing aids, the medicine list has the stamp of polypharmacy and the heart has been decorated with a couple of stents, we finally turn to spirituality to save us from the miserable slow winding down road of body shut down to the cremation pyre or burial ground.

It is this key question, the answer to which the Gita asks you to seek. Western psychology finally stresses mindfulness as a key concept in the treatment of mental health issues, but does not bother to explain the concept behind the practice. It does not even define the 'who' who is doing the mindfulness practice. Sadly, allopathic medicine does not even accurately define 'life 'because it cannot define what makes us alive.

The Bhagavad Gita does. Search in the Bhagavad Gita, not in the wrong places. Like Prabhupada is in his own inimitable manner says the hogs who are revelling in their own faeces have no time to enjoy delicious sweets made of **ghee**. (clarified butter) He writes in the purport (B.G.2:1): 'Material compassion, lamentation and tears are all signs of the ignorance of the real self.

It is like crying for the dress of a drowning man, not the man himself'. Prabhupada says: 'Compassion for the dress of a drowning man is senseless. A man who has fallen into the ocean of nescience (ignorance) cannot be saved by simply rescuing his outward dress- the gross material body.' Compassion for the soul (the real entity) is possible only when we realize who we truly are. This realization can only come, if we start on the journey to make ourselves eligible to receive the required knowledge.

CHAPTER 3

BECOMING ELIGIBLE TO SEARCH THE RIGHT KNOWLEDGE STEP 1: KARM YOGA

How does one make oneself eligible to receive the right knowledge? When one's mind is already stuffed with beliefs and conditioned to think in a certain way, it is difficult to do so.

A cleansing process is essential.

Consider pots filled with water as an analogy for the mind.

There are 3 pots. One with pure clear water, one with slightly muddy water and one contaminated with garbage and leaves. Put these out in the bright noon sunlight and check the reflection of the sun. The sun reflects brightest from the surface that has no dirt, so it is with our minds.

The famous saying goes, the mind is the mirror of our soul, but in the present times for most people the mind (moods, thoughts) itself feels so difficult to control, the soul feels like a universe away. One may agree to believe that each of us is a soul. That is the immortal being Krishna is referring to when he puts the question to Arjuna: 'Who is the slayer? Who is the slain?'

We are all embodied souls.

All world religions tell you this, but the knowledge is similar to what we would have for chocolate, had we had never tasted it: We would know it's color, shape, consistency and smell and all the knowledge that our senses of perception and previous learning gave us but the aha melt in the mouth sensation that all the famous chocolatiers lure us with, we will never know.

How do we start the journey of discovering the delicious stuff? Experience the sensation of bliss that the sugar gives without having the sugar in the mouth?

Again it is a process of knowledge coupled with a belief in the Supreme Consciousness (Krishna, Allah, Adonai, God, Waheguru, Ahura Mazda), whatever name you wish to use.

Because if one agrees to believe that one is an embodied soul, it follows that one also believes that there is a Person/Force out there who makes the sun shine and the moon look glorious, the wheat grow and the rivers flow. Even a small factory cannot function without an owner and manager. So how can one complacently suppose that the macrocosm and the microcosm does?

If you agree that there is a supreme controller of the complete set up managing the show, it is logical to show our gratitude. So, at our home, Jacob, every Friday night we faithfully light the Shabbat candles and say the two-minute prayer.

We remember the Supreme Controller again next Friday. The Gita asks us to remember Him moment to moment in whatever form or name you wish.

But is that possible?

Is it possible to still the mind?

Arjuna also shares the same perspective with Krishna (B.G.6:33) He says 'For the mind is restless, turbulent, obstinate and very strong, O Krishna and to subdue it, I think is more difficult that controlling the wind'.

Sri Krishna teaches Arjuna about Karm Yog as a starting point on how to quieten the mind.

What is Karm Yog? This is a specific process outlined in the third chapter of the Bhagavad Gita. This must not be confused with breathing practices and body postures (**Hatha Yog**) The meaning of the word Yog is to unite, sadly a beleaguered word, flaunted around carelessly.

And what is Karm Yog? How does this practice affect our minds in a beneficial way? Does practicing this remove a roadblock to happiness? Yes. it will, but it is not a pill. It is a process, difficult early on in practice, but brings satisfaction once mastered.

Srila Prabhupada Bhaktivedanta writes in his purport (B.G.3:3) 'Religion without philosophy is sentiment or sometimes fanaticism, while philosophy without religion is mental speculation'. The Gita neither preaches a religion, nor is it only a philosophy. It imparts knowledge which is transcendental. The term **'transcendental'** is an apparently confusing word until you crack the real meaning. But then like the water in the pot, your mind has to be clear to get it.

How does one get one's mind to that level? Karm Yog is required. Karm Yog is the kindergarten class to make the mind ready to go to that level. Sadly, today much of the world's population at this time does not know about Karm – Yog or may think it a waste of time. Because it is more hip to get a quick fix.

Many teenagers and young adults come to the clinic with their self-diagnosed diagnosis- 'I have ADHD'-attention deficit hyperactivity disorder (classified in the DSM-5 psychiatric guidelines as a neurodevelopmental disorder) There is the magic drug 'Vyvanse' The university authorities are also in abeyance. They grant special concessions, more time for assignments and tests for the person who has ADHD. My job is simple- write the prescription and fill the form, submerge the symptom and ignore the root cause. Karm Yog does not fit into my prescription pad.

The woman in her twenties tells me she has OCD-obsessive compulsive disorder (DSM-5 obsessive compulsive and related disorders). I wrote her a prescription for escitalopram. That is indeed an effective drug. She will be profusely thanking me in a few weeks. Her husband has a video game addiction (DSM-5 Internet gaming disorder). Counselling is a very expensive, not so quick fix for this.

For those who can eschew the quick fix there is Karm-Yog as a starter. But what is this Karm Yog? You ask. To climb the hill, we need to start at the bottom – Karm Yog is the trail to the top. Karm is any activity be it thought, speech or physical work that I do with the awareness that I am doing it. For example, breathing, eating and walking are Karm, beating of the heart, digestion is not. Activity implies motion, motion permanently stops only when the heart stops. Till then, the embodied being cannot relinquish Karm, except in deep sleep (because the mind is in silent mode, then) or in meditation. To do any Karm the "I" sense has to be present, so it is even in a dream. Animals, birds and plants are not capable of Karm. That is why human life is deemed unique and precious.

Thought is mental activity, speech is verbal activity and action is physical activity.

Any action requires 5 factors: Human body and mind, sense of doership "I", life force and an external factor, about which we will talk later.

So, what are the constituents of action? **Karanam** – the instrument (senses, mind and body), **Karm** – the work itself and **Karta** – the doer.

What motivates action? **Jnanam-** knowledge, **Jneyam** – the object of the knowledge and **Parijnata-** the knower.

A simple example to illustrate the above terms would be, I know (knower) chocolate ice-cream tastes good (knowledge), so why do I not eat some chocolate ice-cream (object of knowledge). Next steps will be directed to the fridge.

Karm- Yog is just notching Karm to a higher level, linking it to a higher ideal. The one who is not a Karm- yogi is a **kripana** – a miser. It is your choice which one you wish to be.

Karm Yog is the process that can clear and detoxify the mind, enabling it to receive the knowledge of the Gita..

It is the spiritual paradigm of working in the world, where one becomes free of the fear of unknown consequences. The entrepreneur may head a successful venture, yet may not be able to get a good night's sleep worrying about future outcomes. He does enjoy the benefits of his success but in spite of being so is not at peace. Karm Yog lets success bind you with a golden chain, not an iron one.

Karm Yog generates spiritual energy/wealth. In contrast to being obsessed with happiness and unhappiness, one moves ahead to regard both with equanimity.

Karm Yog makes one think and work in an efficient manner, does not promote lethargy. It promotes empathy.

When one is a Karm yogi one works with happiness, not for happiness. One works with contentment, not for contentment. So back to dissecting what Karm Yog means:

Karm becomes Karm- Yog when any Karm (as defined earlier) has the following characteristics:

1. The Karm (action) is done with a sense of equanimity **(samatva buddhi)** abandoning all attachment to success or failure. It is done without getting agitated, not prompted by ego, anger or confusion.
2. It is based on what is right and what needs to be done, not what I like or dislike, **(swardhama buddhi)**. Whether it is fun or no fun, we do it with the same zeal, The common example here will be 'my exams are approaching, it feels more fun to watch a cricket or football match, but right now I should be studying so that I what I devote my time too'
3. The Karm is dedicated to a higher goal **(sampurna buddhi)**. Do it not only for your welfare but for the welfare of others too. The Karm is performed not for your ego, nor to get praise from other people. Examples of the opposite: I wrote this amazing book. I really deserve to bag the Booker prize or at least get shortlisted for it. If I see more patients today in less time, I will get more money for my time, it really does not matter if the patient is attended to properly or not. Most of the time we ask ourselves whenever faced with a task, assignment, or work 'what is in it for me, if I am not benefited, why should I do it.' This trend of thinking comes, because we see ourselves as individuals and not as part of a whole. The father asks

his teenager to clean the basement, no response, then shouts, after fifteen minutes screams. Half an hour later, the basement is still littered with popcorn and chips. The son is still debating why I should be doing the cleaning? The son does not see himself as part of the whole, that cleaning the house as a joint responsibility, not only the father's as all the family lives here. The son sees himself as an individual entitled to live in the house because of his birth, but not as part of a unit.

4. There is no attachment to the result of the action (**Asanga buddhi**). One can plan for the result, yet not be attached to it. One has a right to perform the action, but is not entitled to the result. Any attachment, positive or negative, is a cause of bondage. A pharmacist from India needed to do her licensing exam in Canada to be able to practice. She had all the knowledge, but when she attempted the exams, she failed. This happened repeatedly for a second and a third time till at the fourth year she could not even bring herself to fill the application for the exam. When the next exam date was announced, she postponed the attempt as she was convinced she would fail again. Her time was spent more on focussing on the result, than on the preparation. Focus on the result, endure the stress which is attendant.

5. Offer the result of the Karm to the Supreme Consciousness (**Prasad buddhi**). You do agree he is your Maker and your ultimate Boss. The ordinary person looks to the world for his happiness, projects into the future (anticipation of the planned vacation) or reminisces about the past (good old days). In **Prasad buddhi** our attention is focused on the present.

Karm Yog changes our attitude so that even if an undesirable result occurs, we do not get agitated. It changes our perspective so that we can look at failure and success both with equanimity (there is a difference between equanimity and indifference).

At the lowest level, a person does not do anything. Little better: does something good but with selfish motive, better: does something good but without selfish motive. Best: doing everything with Karm -Yog

The secret to success to becoming a Karm- yogi is being aware all the time whether or not you are able to do all the 5 check marks, day in and day out and ask yourself, if you are progressing.

As you progress, you begin to contemplate more, react less, choose your words more carefully, ego trips decrease, obsessions and aversions disappear. This combination of action and contemplation has one incredulous side effect. Work is no longer work. Work is a flower placed at the altar of the One who made you in the first place Work is no longer a stone tied around your neck. Stress and burnout become irrelevant terminology.

CHAPTER 4

BECOMING ELIGIBLE TO SEARCH THE RIGHT KNOWLEDGE STEP 2: DAILY SADHANA

What is daily **sadhana** and how does it help to search for the right knowledge along with Karm yog?

It helps in the quieting of the mind and in the acquisition of spiritual knowledge. Spiritual knowledge in contrast to material knowledge is cyclical. (Material knowledge is linear, something that grows as we know more and more) but spiritual knowledge needs cyclic repetition till assimilated. Sadhana **is** a daily spiritual practice.

Set time aside for it daily. As *Keshava Swami says on YouTube: The Ranveer Show episode 347*: Become a member of the 5 am club: get up an hour or two before sunrise to do sadhana. In his words 'when the archer is about to release an arrow, the first thing that the archer does is to pull back. When we pull, although it seems that you are going further away from your target, it allows you to generate power, it allows you to direct and release for maximum impact' If you want maximum impact in your life, you can liken sadhana to a bowman pulling the arrow back. We disconnect from the world and connect with our original identity. The member of the 5 am club is ready for his worldly activity at 8 am.

Swami Mukundananda (YouTube: The Ranveer Show Hindi 70) gives this analogy: If you mix milk with water, it dissolves in it. Its identity is changed, just like our minds are affected by the news and life experiences that we get. But if we set the milk aside for some time away from water, it will turn into curd and the curd can be churned into butter. Now if you put the butter into water, it will not dissolve. It can now challenge the water.

Our minds can also challenge the onslaught of outside happenings and be victorious, if we devote an hour or two daily to separating the mind (milk) from the outside world (water). In that precious time, what do you do? Give knowledge to the ignorant mind, focus to the scattered mind and a deep cleansing if the mind is excessively muddied.

Use the techniques outlined in The Bhagavad Gita to calm the restless mind and increase focus, without which the mind like the milk cannot transform into the gold of butter. It could chanting a mantra or concentrating on the breath.

Mantra – man (mind) tra (free). A grouping of words spoken repeatedly with full concentration, without the mind wandering into the rest of the day or into the past or future. You say the same mantra daily, do not change. The time before sunrise is the best. Even in the Islamic tradition great importance is given to the morning prayer to be performed specifically before dawn.

A few rules need to be observed. Sit erect. Sit in the same place every day at the same time, not after food, not when you are sleepy. The place should be clean and not used for any other purpose. The seat must be comfortable, but not so comfortable that you doze off. The body needs to remain motionless with a 'no entry' sign pasted on the door of the mind. If a thought does enter, do not look at it, but let it pass. Do not react to it. Immediately after your daily sadhana, do not shake off the side effects- but gradually slide into the rest of the day.

Listening to spiritual literature/musical compositions, studying spiritual literature or reciting a prayer in this golden hour are also components of daily sadhana.

One needs to structure and follow this spiritual exercise daily with discipline. It is not an arduous journey. Sri Krishna is a great teacher, compassionate and caring. And when you sing His name, he imparts special tuition to you.

When the mind is primed by Karm – Yog, and we do the daily morning practice, our thoughts change. When the thoughts change, the convictions change. When convictions change, character building occurs: **Swabhava** is the Sanskrit word for one's internal mental composition Take the help of the Bhagavad Gita to lead you up to your goal, just like the pole vaulter soars into space with the help of the pole and lands victorious on the other side of the sand pit, much further away than he could have ever done by himself.

CHAPTER 5

PROGRESSING TO THE NEXT STEP: THE CONCEPT OF SEVA

We make a living by what we get but we make a life by what we give. *(Keshava Swami on YouTubeTRS 347)* The concept **of seva** is linked to Karm – Yog. It strengthens the effect of the daily morning practice (sadhana).

Mother Teresa said 'The hands that help are holier than the lips that pray 'The Gita says' let worship not be an act (daily prayer) let every act of yours be a worship of the Lord'

Seva is much more than volunteering. But volunteering can be a starting point. **Seva** roughly translates into the English word service, but incompletely. Seva is service to other living beings as a principle of life.

To do justice to the word we need to understand much more. In Chap 2 Sri Krishna tells Arjuna 'Neither are you the slayer nor are they the ones who will be slain. 'And asks 'So, who are you?'

Who is the real you? Is it the body? Is it the mind? Vedic literature goes to great lengths to put forth logical, sound arguments to prove that we are neither. We can either choose to study the Vedic tomes or simply believe the Bhagavad Gita. (B.G.5:4) Both paths lead to the same conclusion. So, if we are not the body and not the mind, what are we?

Because of our conditioned thinking, we identify ourselves as man, woman or the, new classification LGBTQ, white, brown or other colour, tall, short or in-between and add the tag of the nation/religion we were born in to further solidify our sense of identity. But our identity is not just a thought, just as the thought of a flower is not a flower and thinking about water will not quench my thirst. The I that we think we are is not the true I.

The true 'I' is the consciousness, referred to as **atma** in sanskrit or the self, the entity which itself does not do any act but in whose presence the body and mind functions akin to a movie screen on which we see the film. The screen itself is blank, but without the screen there is no movie. Without the atma (consciousness), the mind does not function, the body rots. The atma/self is the resident in the city of nine gates (the body) and pervades it. The decay of the body is initiated by its exit.

The ignorant person identifies with the body, the enlightened person knows he is the I 'living in the city of nine gates'. Sri Ramakrishna, who is considered an **avatar** of Krishna and the guru of Swami Vivekananda says people can be compared to fish in the ocean. The smart ones know the world can lure them away from their soul, so they keep alert and away from the fisherman's net, the second type get caught, realise the danger and jump out before it is too late and the third variety lie without disturbance not knowing they are going to be fried and dead. After death there is no redemption, the time to act is now and here.

The real 'I' is hidden from view, we can only realize it through the instrument of the mind by applying the knowledge and practices given in the Gita. Other traditions like Buddhism, Sikhism and Sufism also have similar teachings One needs to choose according to one's inclination.

Do **seva,** it increases your bank balance for the life after death, the life after this life. We plan for many uncertain things that may not happen, but we do not plan for the most inevitable event of our life, that is death. Sadly, in this day and age people do not even contemplate on what happens after death. There is a book called the *Garuda Purana* which exquisitely details the horrors of the different hells that the non believer goes through. We talk about the increasing number of suicides, but the suffering one undergoes after the suicide is far worse than the one preceding it (as per the *Garud Purana*). Unfortunately, the suicdee cannot communicate with us in detail. We are either terrified by ghosts or we simply say prove it. Some facts and stories cannot be not proved to folks with limited senses- It gets conveniently lumped into mythology.

Seva: - because I am not alone, I am part of the whole.

- because I am the server, not the enjoyer. I am here on this earth not to enjoy, but for a purpose.

- because I need to break the ego trip which is a start point for the journey of sorrow.

Jacob, you will say this is a handful or just say nothing at all. People generally have an impression that becoming spiritual means withdrawing from the world. A sort of lethargic, inactive person: someone who left the race behind. Nothing could be farther from the truth. You can be as zealous, as enthusiastic, as energetic as anyone else and yet be spiritual. You can be totally immersed in your career and yet be detached from it or you can be physically in a cave and be mentally in the marketplace.

Read the autobiography of the author of the *Bhagavad Gita as it is*. Other inspirational books are *My journey home by Radhanath Swami* and *My lessons with the Himalayan Masters by Swami Rama*.

No long arduous journey to the Himalayas is required for the discovery process. One does not need to hand in his or her resignation letter and go for **Sanyas**. (retirement) Just choose to be a Karm yogi and serve other living beings, human or non human. Do not wait for an opportunity to come to you to do good, go searching for it.

CHAPTER 6

CONTINUING THE RIGHT STEPS WITH THE RIGHT ATTITUDE:
Vivek, Bhava, Sankalpa. Shraddha, Sharangati, Dharma

The practices enumerated in the previous chapters (**Karm Yog, sadhana and seva**) if done consistently over a period of time do bring about a feeling of being livelier, less cynical, less stiff upper lip, less preoccupied with stuff that is not world altering. If one comes from a theistic tradition, where worship of the Lord is relegated to formal prayers, one will encounter a sharp difference.

To understand this, one must know that the Vedic literature of which the Bhagavad Gita is a part is set in a different temporal and spatial zone. The land was bountiful, the arts, architecture, science and culture flourished, the people had no shortage of food, clothing and shelter. The royalty wore ornaments of gold with precious stones and lived in palatial buildings There were debates on what was true and what was untrue, not sermons. The Bhagavad Gita and other Vedic literature are replete with stories, magnificent and spectacular, God (**Avatar of God, Sri Krishna**) is not portrayed as someone to be obeyed or feared. He dances and plays music.

Knowledge is shared, choices are presented and contemplation is requested. The knowledge presented in this priceless book goes beyond the realm of formal religion, that most people practice. It teaches: Get the right knowledge with the right attitude and then progress to the right action.

Get to know that the real source of happiness lies within you. Our senses search for happiness outside us because they are programmed to do so and the mind follows helplessly in the futile search for fulfillment.

The story of the *Princess of Kashi. (Adapted from the YouTube video by Swami Priyananda)* might make the above sentence make more sense:

Once in a kingdom in ancient India, a play was to be staged during a court function on one occasion. In the play, one of the roles was that of a little girl who was the princess of Kashi (a city in ancient India) The 5-year-old prince played the role of the princess, as his mother could not get any one else whom she felt would be appropriate. So, the prince was dressed as a princess and the play was staged. The boy looked so cute that the queen said "make a painting." So, the court painter made a portrait of the boy dressed as a princess, titled and dated it appropriately. Fifteen years passed. The prince was now quite grown up and doing all the princely activities. One day when he was exploring the palace, he went into the underground storage and discovered this painting. He cleaned off the dust and looked at the date. "She seems to be nearly the same age as me". He fell in love with the girl in the picture "this is the princess I want to marry. Unless I can have this princess, I will never be happy again." But he was shy and could not tell his parents, the king and the queen. They noticed something was wrong with their son. He seemed to be moping around and did not seem to be interested in anything.

Finally, a wise minister went and asked him" What ails you prince? You can confide in me."

The prince replied "What can I tell you? I am in love"

"That is very good. Who's she?"

"She is the princess of Kashi"

"Where did you meet her?"

"I have not met her I have only seen her picture"

"Very well. Where is the picture?"

"If it is down in the storage I will show it to you. It is a very old picture. It is dated fifteen years ago."

So, the prince took the minister down into the cellar and showed him the painting. The minister saw the painting and said "Prince, you need to sit down" He told him the story of the drama, how the prince was dressed as the princess and the making of the portrait "The princess is none other than you, yourself."

The desire of the prince to seek the princess for marriage disappeared- the princess of Kashi did not exist apart from him.

For us, too, the princess of Kashi (happiness) exists in us. When we will actually know, the hankering and desire to search outwards will cease.

But like in the story, a guide (the minister) has to show the way.

One needs to work with both mind and heart, intellect by itself is inadequate. The process requires mental spring cleaning, decluttering and rearrangement The daily practice outlined in the previous chapters is essential.

The daily spiritual practice, seva and Karm-Yog are also essential for developing the qualities of **Vivek, Bhava, Sankalp, Shraddha** and **Sharangati**.

Vivek: The power of being able to discern right from wrong, to choose wisely in different situations in life, what facts to believe and which to discard. When we are able to do so, the chances of being misled up the wrong path or making wrong decisions in life decreases.

Bhava: What is your EQ (emotional quotient) level? Do you feel for people or do you feel unmoved at the sight of others' suffering? Mother Teresa felt the distress of the slum dwellers outside her convent in the city of Calcutta. She spent the rest of her life serving these people. Her distinction is that she chose to serve with love, with affection. Similarly, our relationship with Krishna or whatever form of the Supreme Consciousness we choose to revere needs to be one with feeling, not dry and intellectual.

Shraddha: when you enter the school/college classroom and the physics lecturer enunciates the law of motion or the maths teacher talks to you about the Pythagoras theorem, you agree to listen to them and accept that knowledge. The Gita asks you to do the same: do not believe blindly but at least keep an open mind. Have shraddha for Sri Krishna. Have faith that what He teaches you is good for you.

Sankalpa: the power of determination. How determined are you to get out of the cycle of joy and sorrow, not continue to lick the bottle of honey from outside but actually open and taste it? How determined are you to realise your true identity? It is only when this becomes a real hunger, will you try to satiate it.

Sharanagati: Surrender. The word surrender has a martial connotation: frustration, failure, what suffering will I undergo at the hands of the enemy, but *Chaitanya Charan Das in his podcast on the concept of surrender in the Bhagavad Gita* turns the whole idea around. Surrender to God/Supreme consciousness is in 3 stages: First asking God to give you the intelligence to do what is right, when you do not know what is the right thing to do. Intelligence to decide what is the right course of action. Second, surrender to God/Supreme Consciousness when your impulses are so strong that you know the habit that you are doing (for example smoking, alcohol) is harmful to you but yet cannot resist them. The third stage of surrender means doing the will of God with whatever gifts he has endowed you with. As the Bible also says, 'Thy will shall be done' Use our gifts to do the will of God. (from *Three understandings of surrender in the Bhagavad Gita – Chaitanya Charan Das*)

Sharangati also implies that I agree that for whatever I consume or obtain, the provider is the Supreme. For example, one may say, 'I cooked a delicious dish of potatoes and cauliflower, I made the recipe.' but you neither made the potato germinate or the cauliflower grow. You acknowledge that it is the benevolence of the Supreme that the delicious food is on the table.

Sharanagati is possible only when one has humility and complete trust in the Supreme Consciousness, knowing He will do what is appropriate for us. It is then possible for us to give up our bad tendencies just as diabetic gives up eating sugar knowing it is harmful for him. With humility, one surrenders and serves, but unlike the martial surrender, the result is immense joy and peace.

Swami Mukundananda has a different take on this subject in his book *Spiritual secrets of Hinduism*. He states that Sharanagati means not only accepting the will of God when faced with a problem, but also not getting disturbed when things continue not going your way.

He tells the story of a man who reached the edge of the forest and had to cross a river. The man prayed to God to give him wings to fly across. Nothing happened, he kept walking and then prayed for a boat. Still nothing happened, so he kept walking along the river's edge. Finally, he came to the bridge and could cross over to the other side of the river.

The biggest roadblock to Sharanagati is pride. Swamiji says in his book: give up the pride that you are the doer, even the pride that you have surrendered.

All the above qualities help one develop a deeper insight into life so that one's perspective on work, people and situations changes. These will remain the same, the lens through which you view them changes. Your concept of you changes: you are not body, not mind. The body and mind are the containers of the real you.

But these containers need to be cleaned, purified so that you can progress in your journey to search for happiness.

CHAPTER 7

THE RIGHT ATTITUDE NEEDS A CLEAN CONTAINER: THE THREE GUNAS

What do I mean by calling the body and mind, the container of the soul?

Let me take the help of *Swami Sarvapriyananda* again. In one of his YouTube videos. He refers to a sci-fi book where one alien is talking to another after visiting Earth

Alien 1 "What did you see there"

Alien 2 "A lot of people driving their cars around. They fill them up and spend a lot of time in them"

Alien 1: "Looks like they are very busy and occupied with cars"

Yes, the car has become more than a vehicle to get from Place A to Place B. It can be the Lexus of a status symbol or the Ferrari of a teenager's dream.

Each of us is the driver within the car of the human body, and like the alien's depiction, we keep very busy with this very visible entity that we are given, to the extent that it is a major part of our identity.

The body, mind. and intellect are however just the containers that house the **atma**/consciousness/self. The car and the driver of the car are separate and different.

If you have made the journey up to this chapter, you are surely in agreement. The task is now how to actually use this car of the human body and mind in the service of the driver (the **atma/**consciousness) instead of glossing over that it is indeed a Lexus and not a KIA.

For starters, put good food inside. Our bodies are made up of what we eat. Eat junk and our bodies become junk. The body in Vedic terminology is called **anna maya kosha**. It is one of the envelopes surrounding the **atma** and the one that is visible to the eye.

Anna: means food. **Kosha** means envelope. The food we eat gets transformed into our muscles, tissues and blood. The quality of the food even determines how one feels: sluggish, slow, vs light, active and alert. If the pot (container of the **atma**) is full of dirt, the inner contents will be muddy. So how do we make our bodies vibrant, our skin glow and the mind clear.? Eat **Sattvic** food for starters.

What do I mean by **Sattvic** food? What does the term **'Sattvic'** mean anyway? **Sattva, Rajas and Tamas** are the three Gunas.

Understanding the concept of the three Gunas is essential to the knowledge that the Gita offers.

In Chapter 14, Sri Krishna says 'Everyone has some type of attributes or qualities to which one is inclined to'. He describes 3 types. The term used in the Bhagavad Gita for these three facets of personality/attributes is **Guna**, which interestingly translates also to rope. The rope that binds the **atma**/self/consciousness and prevents it from reaching its eternal home with its Maker. Only **Sattva Guna** is kinder than the others. In **Sattva Guna**, the rope starts unravelling.

This concept of defining a person's personality fits well with the concept of a human (**Jiva**) having three components:(This is a simplified breakup for the purpose of this book)

1. **Stul sharir/annamayakosha:** the gross body, the one that is visible to us.
2. **Sukshma Sharir** which is commonly termed mind, subtle body.
3. **Adhayamantar/atma** consciousness, spirit.

The consciousness/**atma**/soul is the essential me and is ensconced in the gross and subtle body. Though the soul itself has no attributes, like the air that carries a particular smell, it takes up the hue of the mind. I can be a good person, an active person or a bad person, depending on which Guna predominates within me. The soul bound with the gross and subtle body forgets who it really is, like an actor who has forgotten that he is an actor and becomes the character he plays. He gets entrapped in the fortress of **Prakriti** and continues to do so, birth after birth.

What is meant by **prakriti?** For want of a better word, we can define it as material nature or all that we experience through our sense organs and mind. The fourteenth chapter of the Gita gives a detailed description of it. All of what we see and experience in this material world is **Maya**. So though each of us is essentially a tiny particle of consciousness, being inside the body, we are entangled with **prakriti,** which makes us dance as a puppeteer does with the puppet on strings through the three Gunas. These decide our mental attributes. The three modes function like puppeteer strings. We are the puppets strung by 3 threads, but we do not know. When a drunken person is in jail, the outsider knows he is imprisoned, but the drunkard who is, knows not.

The enlightened person is one who has been able to break the control of the Gunas on him or her, though he continues to remain embodied. **Prakriti** cannot play cat and mouse with this person any more. He knows that sorrow and joy are both impermanent and chooses not to come under their sway. So are pleasure and pain and the other dualities that we battle with through each lifetime.

The Gita describes the three Gunas as

Sattva: light, knowledge, goodness. Sattva is defined as the Guna (state of the body and mind) where goodness, equanimity and peace prevail. When one is in Sattva Gun, knowledge flows from in from the outside world and the mind responds with intellect and intuition.

Rajas: action, motion, tendency to quick anger. Rajas is where the person has intense activity, he/she probably has a whirlwind of thoughts going on in the mind. Rajogun breeds selfishness, sees division – mine and not mine. As the rajasic component of one's personality increases, so does the hankering for greater sense enjoyment, more material acquisition and anticipation of prestige and recognition in society. This is the current trend in today's society: work hard, achieve wealth and status and you are considered successful. Modern society is therefore compared to a duck in water: smooth and graceful above, but paddling like crazy below the water.

Tamas: darkness, absence of activity, laziness, tendency to be morose, delusion. The most appropriate word would be inadvertence **(pramadh)** It can be further described as a state of carelessness, unawareness, confusion: the intellect is not functioning in the correct manner. Tamas is where the mind, like the crocodile in the zoo or riverbank, lies in a state of sloth or is completely deluded. When the mind is tamasic, the body gets tamasic desires. The body says 'I am tired 'even though the person needs to work. The mind tells the body to sleep even though the intellect had decided it was important to get up early. The person with a tamasic mind sees what is wrong as right and what is right as wrong. Instead of progressing, he gradually degrades himself. Sri Ramakrishna describes the state of tamas: There are three types of fish: 1. Certain types of fish never get caught in the net. 2. some get caught and struggle to get free. 3. The third type gets caught but do not even know that they are caught. The third variety is in a state of tamas.

The following story further Illustrates the concept of the three gunas. The story of the three robbers. (*adapted from the YouTube video by Swami Sankarananda: The 3 Gunas and the story of the three Robbers*)

Once in ancient India, there was a traveller who had many jewels and precious stones with him. He had to pass through a dense forest to reach his home. In the forest, three robbers accosted him, robbed him of his jewels, beat him up and then tied him to a tree. One of the robbers said "let us kill him."

Another said "why should we taint our hands with his blood? Just leave him tied up, a tiger or lion will probably eat him up" So they left.

After a short while, the third robber approached the bruised and beaten-up traveller, freed his ropes and told him. "I will show you the way safely out of the forest."

So, the two of them walked along till the traveller's village was in sight. Grateful to the third robber, the traveller invited him to his home. The robber declined "Sir, the forest edge determines my limits, I cannot trespass it."

The traveller is the **atma**/soul. The home in the village represents his final destination.

The three robbers are the three gunas who rob the jewels and tie him up.

The first robber, who wants to kill the traveller, represents Tamas which deadens the mind. An overload of Tamas is clinical depression.

The second robber represents Rajas, full of action, not that evil but not that good either.

The third robber, Sattva Guna, is the one who shows the way out of the forest to the traveller.

The forest represents life in the material world. As long as we remain in the forest, we cannot reach our home, cannot realize our true identity. The good thing about the Sattva Guna is that like the third robber, it can show us the way out. When the traveller is free of the three robbers, he reaches home. When the mind crosses all the three states, beyond all three gunas, it realizes that he actually is just consciousness.

Sattva Guna itself cannot bring about self realization, but it can lead us there, lead us out of the forest and to the village that is our home.

All three modes are present within us. Modes fluctuate through life. One mode may predominate over others at different times of our lives. Our mental make up is determined by which mode is predominant within us. We need to keep the three Gunas in balance with the predominance of Sattva and progressive diminution of Tamas.

As which Guna predominates in you, so do you act:

The story of the 3 hat seller brothers:

The first brother is in Tamogun: He sits under a tree and the monkeys come and take away his wares. He gets despondent, goes to the pub and drinks his sorrows away.

The second brother is in Rajogun: He sits under a tree and the monkeys come and take away the hats he is going to market to sell. He gets angry, shouts at monkeys, gets tired and goes away.

The third brother is in Sattvagun: He sits under a tree and the monkeys come and take away his hats: He wears his own hat, stands in front of the monkeys, makes a face and throws his hat down. The monkeys follow suit. The third brother collects his wares and goes to market to sell.

This may sound like a very simplistic tale but the truth is if you are in sattva, there is an increase in clarity, being in the 'feeling good state' and conditioned to obtaining knowledge, if you are predominantly rajasic there is much hankering and attachment whilst tamas gives you a dollop of misery and lethargy.

Only by being in Sattva, can one transcend sorrow. Tamo bandages sorrow. If one is predominantly in Rajasic mode but lives in a tamasic atmosphere for example, the family members are tamasic, the sorrow becomes worse. Tamas lowers the level of knowledge: It is like driving in the mountains at night with the headlights turned off. A person in Tamogun cannot help himself. He needs someone to help him. A Rajasic person can help himself and transcend to a predominantly Sattvic state. In Sattvagun, there is inspiration to act, in Rajogun there is motivation to act. In Tamogun there is instigation to act.

Modes also fluctuate through the time of the day: The day (circadian rhythm) is also divided into sattvic, rajasic and tamasic periods: Between midnight at 8 am Sattva is prominent, between 8 am and 4 pm, Rajogun is active, between 4 pm and midnight is when Tamas predominates.

If Tamogun is absent, we cannot sleep. Tamogun can be used positively to rest. If Rajo Gun is absent, we cannot work. The mode of sattva conditions one to happiness, the mode of rajas to fruitive actions, while tamas brings distress and laziness.

The three gunas within each human being are in a state of flux: when one predominates, the others decrease. It could be 40: 30: 30 percent of time or 60: 30: 10 or 40: 40: 10. When a person sits quietly in a prayer meeting and listens attentively he is Sattva Guna, if he dozes off, he is in Tamogun. If he is fidgety and keeps checking his watch, he is in Rajogun. Rajo can go either into Sattva or Tamo. By suppressing Tamo and Rajo, Sattva arises, when we try to keep our mind quiet, Sattva increases. When the mind chants, it is given an activity that quietens it.

In Vedic literature the analogy of the rope vs the snake is often cited. The Rajasic person sees the rope as a snake. The Sattvic person sees the rope is not a snake. The Tamasic person is so fearful he does not want to look at the object at all.

The knowledge of the Gunas is also compared to worldly knowledge as 'When one goes out in the rain, one needs an umbrella not a crown'

The three Gunas are also compared to 3 gloves: the gloves of the surgeon, wicket keeper and a boxer. One can thread a needle easily only with the surgical gloves- Sattva.

Sattvagun can also be compared to a smoke surrounding the fire- fire is easily visible.

Rajogun: dust covering a mirror. Dust needs to be removed before the mirror can be used.

Tamogun: fetus in a womb, much work needs to be done before the soul can be delivered.

In Sattva one is more conscious of consciousness. In Tamas one is not. Sattva synergises one's energies with a higher nature, Rajas with active work, Tamas breeds sloth.

A Sattvic person considers work as worship, for the Rajasic, work is a means to benefit oneself. The Tamasic person makes others work and gives himself credit.

But for now, back to food.

Sri Krishna (B.G.17:8) says food dear to those in the mode of goodness is juicy, fatty, wholesome and pleasing to the heart. These are whole grains, fruits and vegetables. Protein is amply available through lentils and nuts. Sattvic food is food that is living. The vegetables still have life in them when we cook them. When the life has left the vegetable, it starts rotting. Grains have the potential to sprout if allowed so there is life contained in them.

Food can be considered Sattvic when the person who has prepared it has a good attitude. There is a reference to milk being included in sattvic food, perhaps in that time period, milk production was not linked with animal cruelty and hormone addition as it is now. Fatty foods, as mentioned here, have no connection with animal fat.

So, what are the foods to avoid? Sri Krishna says: foods that are too bitter, or too sour, salty, hot, pungent, dry and burning are dear to those in the mode of passion (Rajas). Such food causes distress, misery and disease. These foods, because of the additional red pepper, cause decreased mucus secretion in the stomach leading to disease. (Purport by Prabhu pada B.G 17:10). When we eat food that is rajasic, the level of animalistic passion, symptoms of attachment, fruitive activity and thirst for acquiring things increase.

The third and worst category is tamasic foods. Food that is prepared more than three hours ago, before being eaten (except **prasadam** from a temple) and food that cannot be offered as **prasad** to the deity in the temple like meat, fish, eggs, frozen foods made with an expiry date fall in this category. Prabhupada writes in his purport (B.G.14:16) 'Slaughtering poor animals is also due to the mode of ignorance. The animal killers do not know that in the future, the animal will have a body suitable to kill them' He bluntly states 'A civilization that guides the citizens to become animals in their next lives is certainly not a human civilization 'He concludes: 'So, indulgence in animal killing for the taste of the tongue is the grossest kind of ignorance. If one indulges in meat eating anyway, it is to be understood that he is acting in ignorance and is making his future very dark'. When the body is fed tamasic food, it wants to lie down as close to earth as possible. An animal in contrast to a human being is guided by instinct, but a tamasic person falls below instinct.

Again, the way to keep it simple to remember:

'Do not eat anything that comes from anything with two eyes and one mouth'

'Decrease your intake of food that is prepackaged in box or bottle or comes with a barcode'

What comes from farm to plate is healthier than what comes from farm to factory to plate.'

Interestingly, medical science also now agrees that Sattvic diet prevents lifestyle disease (*Dr. Sanjay Kalra in Med Talks YouTube video on heart failure, sept 17, 2023*)

In what other ways do the gunas shape our personalities?

In the actions we perform, the choice of what we adore or worship, the austerities we perform and the charity we give. These are termed in Sanskrit as **Daan, Yagna, Tapas and Karm**.

Yagna is worship: everyone has to worship something. The sattvic person worships the Supreme through prayers and work.

The Rajasic person worships Mammon (money and worldly pleasures) and his service is directed accordingly. The Gita (B.G.17:12) says 'But the sacrifice (yagna) performed for some material benefit, or for the sake of pride, O chief of Bharatas, you should know to be in the mode of passion.' Many people will say I pray regularly or daily, but they pray to God with a goal in mind. God is not their goal. Krishna is for the fulfilment of desire, Krishna is not the fulfillment of desire. (*borrowed from Chaitanya Charan Das*)

The tamasic person worships power or illusory pleasures and spends his time getting increasingly entangled in both, till there is no succour. Prabhupada says tamasic yagna produces a demoniac mentality and does not benefit human society.

The word **yagna** also is used for a fire ceremony, sacrifice. Sattvic yagna is also the term used to define an attitude of sacrifice, and dedication. We sacrifice the lower desires for the higher goal. This is five-fold.

1. **Divyangana:** Thanking the deities for providing us with air, water and light. We get these free everyday but do we stop to think and thank the universal power that is providing these to us?
2. **Pitrayagna:** Thanking our previous generations for the knowledge and culture that they have passed on to us. Like the saying goes: Rome was not built in a day. The previous generation has an input into what we have today and we need to acknowledge and thank them for this.
3. **Rishi yagna:** The Vedic scriptures of which the Bhagavad Gita is a very tiny part were given to us by the **Rishis** (enlightened persons/seers). Neither would I be writing this today nor would you be reading it if the Rishis had not provided us with the knowledge. So, we need to acknowledge this and thank them.
4. **Manushya yagna**: caring and sharing for those human beings who are suffering. The haves of the world need to have compassion for the have nots.
5. **Bhutyagna**: respecting other living beings.

The **yagnas** described above can only be performed when one truly believes that he/she is a part of the whole, just as parts of the tree function for the benefit of the whole tree and the hand puts the food in the mouth to nourish the entire body, not only itself.

The world does not exist to serve our individual needs. We are just one tiny part existing with other living beings ensconced in prakriti. The above describes Sattvic **yagna**.

Similarly, charity **(Daan)** can be performed in any of the three modes.

Sattvic Daan is charity given as duty, without expecting anything in return, done intelligently, at the right time, at the right place and to the right person. Charity needs not only money but also energy and time. If we do not share these, these will be lost. Importantly when doing charity, one respects the receiver, the giver feels honoured that he has been given the opportunity to do service to another living being. **Daan** is done as a way of serving God/Supreme Consciousness, not helping people. Whatever God gives me in the way of wealth and fame, I offer it to Him.

Rajasic daan is done hesitatingly, with expectation of return.

Tamasic daan is charity given to the wrong person, at the wrong time and place.

The third category 'Tapas' can also be classified into the three modes but we first need to clearly understand what Tapas is. The next chapter explains.

Karm. Action: Sri Krishna describes 3 different types of action:

Sattvic action is the action that is ethical and worth doing. Action that is free of attachment to the sense of doership, to the action itself and to the result. Action that is free of likes and dislikes, free of attraction and repulsion.

Rajasic action: action which seeks fulfillment of desire, although one has to go through a lot of trouble for it. The person sees himself/herself as the accomplisher, looks for approval/reward for doing the job well, gets frustrated if he does not get the desired result: passing an exam, earning a sum of money or the desired promotion in the corporate world. The person with Rajasic attributes has intense likes and dislikes: I am so attracted to this person that I will go any length to please her. I detest her mother so much that I cannot bear to enter her parent's home.

Tamasic action: that action which is undertaken through delusion, without considering consequences of action, without considering one's capacity to do it well and action that is done recklessly. Ravana in the Ramayana is pretty descriptive of Tamasic thought and action. He kidnaps Sita, the wife of Rama, knowing very well that he is playing with fire and will not let her go even when his whole nation is deluged in a battle. Because of the stubborn desire to own her, he ultimately loses his life.

Our actions may not be sattvic all the time. Some may be rajasic, some may be tamasic depending on which Guna predominates within us.

If I find that most of my actions are rajasic, then rajasic Guna is predominant. Reviewing and evaluating one's actions and making an effort to preserve the Sattvic actions as well as transform the Rajasic and Tamasic actions into Sattvic is also part of spiritual practice. Doing this practice regularly and with determination increases the predominance of Sattva in one's self.

The following activities increase predominance of Sattva Gun:

1. Arising early in the morning.
2. Daily **Japa** (chanting of holy names)/meditation/prayer.

3. **Pranayama** (part of hatha yoga, involving breathing techniques). Focussing on one's breath also invokes Sattva gun by shifting attention from quiet mind to the 'I' within.
4. Living close to nature.
5. Avoiding being judgemental, controlling or fearful.
6. Being present in the now.
7. Having an association of good people.
8. Eating Sattvic food.

Always be aware of self-talk – is it sattvic, rajasic or tamasic? if a person is predominantly tamasic there is no question of transcendence, evil tendencies have to be destroyed first. To illustrate, if I break the law, I have to go to jail. I do not have a choice. If there is predominance of sattva, there is a possibility to transcend beyond Sattva and achieve the goal of self realization (realizing that one is the consciousness/atma and not mind nor body).

Sattva Guna is like coming to the airport. We come not to live in the airport but to board the flight to our destination. But to take a flight we need to go to the airport first. Sattva is the Guna, that takes one to the airport, from which we can board our flight to self realization.

We have a choice either to continue living in the airport (repeated cycles of birth and death) or board the flight.

CHAPTER 8

MAKING THE CONTAINER DAZZLE: TAPAS

In the previous chapter, I have written about the body being compared to a car/container.

Sri Krishna in the Bhagavad Gita (Chap13) gives the analogy to the concept of mind, body and atma (soul, spirit) as the body being a field of activity, (**ksetram**), soul/atma as the knower of this field (**ksetram- jnam**), the enjoyer (**jiva, purusha**), and nature and nurture (**prakriti**). When I first started reading the Gita, this sounded so vague, I just could not grasp the idea. I went back, studied the commentaries and read the Gita many times over. So finally, after all these years, I understand and can explain the concept to you.

Let us start with the simplified version of the analogy. The field is our body and mind, the ten senses (5 senses of perception 5 senses of action) represent the 10 bulls, The bulls work unceasingly day and night through the field of objects of the senses. The individual soul is the tenant. The five vital airs (**Pranas** respiration, circulation, digestion, reproduction and excretion) are the five labourers. **Prakriti** (nature, nurture and culture: what shapes our personality) is the mistress of the field. She is endowed with the three Gunas. Depending on which Guna is predominant in the field (individual body and mind), the harvest is reaped over time.

If the mistress of the field is predominantly sattvic, seeds of virtue are sowed and a crop of joy is reaped.

Sadly, most tenants (soul/atma/spirit self) get so preoccupied with the field, they forget they have a real home to return to.

The tenant of the field (soul/atma/self) is the knower, the silent witness who is distinct from mind, body and intellect. Just as an iron filing moves in the presence of a magnet, the mind and intellect move and function in the presence of the self. Just as the moon borrows its light from the sun so also the mind and intellect borrow their light from the atma/Self/consciousness The embodied self l is contained in the body, the body is its field of activity. But when the consciousness/atma is embodied (within a body) it forms a consciousness – mind complex (**causal body**) and the world we live in tempts it to enjoy the sensual offerings. The atma forgets who he really is and continues languishing birth after birth in different bodies. He thinks the knowledge that he acquires through the senses and mind is the real knowledge and forgets who he really is.

Sri Krishna says (B.G.13:2)'O Scion of Bharata, you should also understand that I am also the knower of all bodies and to understand this body and its knower is called knowledge. That is my opinion'. But as everything linked with Krishna, there is no dry intellectualism. It is always a matter of linking the heart and brain together. It is not necessary to be intellectual to be spiritual. In the human lifetime Sri Krishna says just acquire these qualities to come closer to realizing your true identity.

1. **Humility:** humility means that one should not be anxious to have the satisfaction of being honored by other people. The material conception of life makes us very eager to get honor from others, but the man who has realized that he

is not this body and mind does not hanker for approval/adoration/recognition from others.
2. **Non-violence:** This term encompasses not only avoidance of physical violence but also not giving any distress to other living beings. (There is an exemption made for the warrior class, those who have to protect the nation)
3. **Tolerance:** When faced with something or some behaviour we do not like, we get agitated. Tolerance is the virtue by which we do not.
4. **Simplicity:** be straightforward in our thinking.
5. **Cleanliness:** This is essential for making progress in spiritual life. The body needs to be kept clean with a daily bath or shower and the mind clean of garbage thoughts. What are the garbage thoughts? Thoughts provoking sorrow and anger, as had happened with these two women in their fifties. They had come to the clinic yesterday for other issues, both broke down and started crying. For the first one, the problem was that her daughter in law had cheated on the lady's son and she had to be asked to leave the matrimonial home. Though the incident had happened a month ago, the woman was still visibly disturbed could not get sleep at night. She kept ruminating about the distress her son was going through. The second lady's situation was even worse. There had been a breakdown of relationships with both the son and daughter-in- law who refused to even let her see her own grandchild. She loudly proclaimed that now only death could relieve her from this misery and she hoped she would die soon. I reminded her that she was only fifty and the average lifespan for women in Canada stretched for a few more decades.

When one is faced with an adverse action by another human being, one can have three responses

a. political: you have hurt me; I will show you/give you back.
b. emotional: you have hurt me, I am miserable.
c. spiritual/intellectual: understand, accept and respond.

Garbage thoughts are also bad/evil thoughts about another person. When one remembers Sri Krishna (or your preferred name be it God, Adonai, Jesus, Allah or Waheguru) constantly, there is no room for garbage thoughts. It works like a vacuum cleaner for the cobwebs of the mind.

6. **Steadfastness:** When one has understood the right path to salvation, which one wishes to pursue, it is important to remain steadfast to the goal.
7. **Self control**: Senses want to perceive and the mind wants to feel. One cannot give a permanent holiday to the senses, but we can feed them the right food. The most difficult by far to control is the sense of taste.
8. **Sense of false ego:** When ones's identity is limited to one's body and mind. One has to remain vigilant and avoid this.
9. **Understanding the distress of birth, death, old age and disease.** When one realises why one goes through this distress repeatedly, one wishes to find a way out of this repeated cycle. There is an entire book, *the Garbo Upanishad* which details the development of the fetus and the travails it goes through in the womb and the process of birth. Similarly, the *Garud Purana* details the suffering that one may go through after death of the body.
10. **Detachment from children, wife and home.** It is easier to drop the 'mine' than the 'me'. So, starting with whom and what you consider yours, care for it or the person but know that it is not an extension of you. To cite an example, your friend has a dog you like very much. One day he says he is going on a trip to Hawaii for a week 'Could you

please keep my dog?' You are overjoyed. The whole week you are busy caring and playing with the dog, but you know it is not yours. Come next week, it will be gone. You do not consider it 'mine'. Your biological relatives are not 'yours' either. They are just co-passengers travelling with you for a short time. Give them love, but do not get needy. Guide them, but do not exercise control. It is interesting too how the concept of mine is so relative. Turning me into mine makes it easier to detach. For example, instead of saying 'I have a headache' you change it to 'my head is hurting'. It is easier to let go of what is mine, than what one considers as me. Look upon your body and mind as instruments. What is connected to the sense of me is more difficult to give up as compared to what one considers as mine. If a robber says your life or your phone, you will readily give up your phone. Use/enjoy what you have but do not get attached to the objects. One of the follies of today's society is that people love objects and use other living beings, instead of the vice versa. The other is the concept of the 'special person in my life' or 'soul mate'. One becomes an adult and seeks complete love and fulfillment in another human being who is as incomplete as themselves. When the biochemical surge subsides, the charm of the relationship ebbs, 'break-up' time occurs and off one goes seeking another stalemate soulmate adventure.

11. **Equanimity:** Equipoised when things are going well and when things are not, not being affected by dualities of hot and cold, poverty and riches, sad events vs happy events. One does not need a vacation to be happy and feel sad when it ends.
12. **Quality of sharing with others:** One who cannot share with others remains miserable. The miser knows only how

to receive, not give, but sometimes that might be their undoing. This short story illustrates.

Once there was a miserly merchant travelling on a boat with 2 other people to cross a river. As per his usual pastime, he took out his purse to count his coins. Unfortunately, one of the coins fell into the water. The merchant jumped out to retrieve the coin, but could not swim. He raised his hands for help. The second passenger shouted 'give me your hand' but the merchant would not, although he was in dire danger of drowning. The boatman told the second passenger 'please rephrase your request, take my hand'. The miser did and was saved.

And how does one acquire these qualities and make the container (mind and body) dazzle? Do **sattvic tapas**.

Though this word is interpreted sometimes as austerity/penance, the root **tap** means to heat so sattvic tapas is a means to purify the mind and body. Tapas is classified as that of the body, speech and mind. Tapas can also be classified according to the three gunas as sattvic, rajasic and tamasic.

Sattvic tapas of the body: keeping our body clean, doing regular exercise, sleeping at the correct times and feeding it sattvic food. A big problem is gut health, many people have problems with bowel movements causing accumulation of **'mal'** toxins in the body. Good gut health translates into a healthy body. There is an excellent discussion on this by *Dr. Pal on the TRS show episode 363. Dr. Pal on Gut health, the mind – food connection and weight loss.*

Sattvic tapas of speech: make your speech sattvic (in the mode of goodness) by avoiding negative talk, not speaking in a manner that agitates the listener beyond his control, ensuring what you speak is truthful and spoken in a manner that is pleasant to the listener. Avoid shouting, it is a waste of sympathetic activity. Avoid judgemental sentences and discriminating verbs. If you need to reprimand someone, do it when you are both by yourselves, not in front of others. First listen and then speak.

Sattvic tapas of mind: I need to use a few Sanskrit words here to be able to convey the complete description.

1. **Saumyatvam:** a mind without duplicity, be straightforward in your thinking.
2. **Manahpasand:** literally translated means happy mind. Manah (mind) pasand (happy). It is our responsibility to keep our mind happy, unconditionally and this needs to be cultivated with effort and faith, because the pleasures of the world cannot eliminate sadness. We can improve only if we improve our mind.
3. **Maunam:** the art of observing the silence of the mind. Mind constantly talks to itself. Most of the talking of the mind is repetitive like an action replay. Sattvic tapas purifies the mind so that it remains in the present moment.
4. **Atmavinagraha.** Thinking should be precise, done when required with avoidance of over thinking or repetitive thinking.
5. **Bhavshamshuddhi:** deal with matters of the world without contamination of hatred, jealousy and pride.

Rajasic tapas: when I do something with my body, speech and mind for an outward result: appreciation, honour by others.

The tamasic person may also do effort but this will be born out of foolish ideas and consequently may bring pain to himself or cause destruction to others. He may practice austerity (tapas) by torturing his body. Prabhupada says that person is only damaging the instrument. When the strings of the Veena (musical instrument) are either too loose or too tight, one cannot make music

When you are in the mode of sattva or goodness you acquire the following qualities and follow these practices to a lesser or greater degree. The greater your score, the higher you are on the rung of the spiritual ladder.

They are 26 and are enumerated as below:

1. **Abhyam:** fearlessness: the presence of purpose makes fear insignificant.
2. **Sattva Samshuddhi:** purification of mind.
3. **Jnana yoga vyavasthiti:** steadfastness in the knowledge of yoga. Some people like to listen to guru (bonafide teacher) for some time, some people like to listen all the time and learn, some dedicate their entire lives to yoga.
4. **Danam:** charity: Develop the mentality of giving. Give regularly, whether big or small. If someone needs more than money, give them that. If one believes that one's joy is in giving to others like Mother Teresa did, one will give.
5. **Dama:** controlling the senses. Marital relationship needs to be more than a sexual relationship.
6. **Yagna:** performance of rituals like chanting, which can be individual (Japa) or community based (sankirtana yajna). This is profoundly life transforming if one is attentive during the ritual.
7. **Svadhyaya:** study of Vedic or other spiritual literature: this is different from academic study. Here one applies the knowledge that one learns to one's emotional, mental and spiritual growth.
8. **Tapas:** austerity. Essentially one is minimising worldly enjoyments and sensual indulgence, accepting material discomforts for increase in spiritual commitment and

preparing for the final exam of death. Like someone quoted, the fewer the things you depend on, the freer you are. You do not have to go to extremes of deprivation. Just feel comfortable even when there is a little discomfort.

9. **Arjavam:** simplicity, uprightness, non crookedness, if we identify the problem correctly, the solution is simple, but if the mind is turbulent, one finds it difficult to do so.
10. **Ahimsa:** non violence to self and others in thought, speech and action. Do not say things negatively.
11. **Satyam:** truthfulness in action, word and thought.
12. **Akrodh:** ability to keep anger in check.
13. **Tyag:** renunciation. Recognizing the things that you do not need and letting go of them. The more distant the journey, the less baggage you have, the happier you will be.
14. **Shanthi.** Tranquility of mind, mind which is least agitated is peaceful. The greater the selfishness, the greater the agitation.
15. **Apaisunam:** aversions to fault finding: no gossip or slander.
16. **Daya:** compassion for all living beings, usually not to all in equal measure.
17. **Alouptvam:** freedom from covetousness, not losing sleep over perishable material things.
18. **Mardavam:** gentleness, the real strong person can be gentle.
19. **Hri:** modesty.
20. **Acapalam:** no fickleness. Use the mind as an instrument. One should be in control of what to think, avoid wasting time on useless thoughts and gossip. Eliminate useless activity in your life. Any thinking, seeking or doing which does not help oneself or others is useless. What is the way to make your mind stop thinking useless thoughts? Remove one toy and give it another. For me, chanting the Hare Krishna mantra instead of letting my mind run

amuck with repetitive thoughts has been a mind-saver. If we can endeavour as above, the mind will be less tired at the end of the day.

21. **Tejas:** boldness, strength, vigor: the positive person exudes a special aura. This particular quality is meant for the men who belong to the warrior class.
22. **Ksama:** forgiveness: only the strong can forgive. This does not mean, not correcting the person or having sleepless nights.
23. **Saucam:** cleanliness of body, mind and speech.
24. **Adrohah:** freedom from hatred.
25. **Dhriti/Titiksha:** Fortitude. Be a big lake where troubles do not cause ripples, bearing the challenges and sorrows in our life without being anxious and grumbling. If I am a little pond and the elephant goes in there will be disturbance. Let your mind be like a great lake that cannot be disturbed by difficulties.
26. **Naiti-manita:** not expecting honor, this applies more to the worker class but may also be interpreted as absence of conceit, superiority complex

You may now question: you have described the good, what about the not – good?

The glaring difference is a person with divine qualities follows the scriptures, the other one does not. Why the scriptures? Because the scriptural knowledge or sastra is far superior to the guidelines for life that we may formulate for ourselves. One cannot lift a bucket while sitting in it. We need perspective from outside us. The Gita says scriptural knowledge is without the four principal defects that are visible in the conditioned soul: imperfect senses, propensity for cheating, certainty of committing mistakes and certainty of being illusioned. It also states that in human society, aversion to understanding the Supreme Consciousness/God/Sri Krishna is the cause of all fall downs. One remains in the realm of ignorance, desire and greed. Prabhupada describes this as a demoniac life and that those having demoniac qualities are the ones who deride the scriptures and do not care to observe the regulations, they disobey the instructions. As he writes in his purport (B.G.16:8) 'Not knowing or believing the scriptures they conclude that there is no controller of the world, that cosmic manifestations arise due to chance material actions and reactions.' 'They have their own theory, that the world has come about in its own way and that there is no reason to believe that there is a God behind it. For them, there is no difference between spirit and matter and they do not accept the Supreme Spirit'.

'They conclude that a child is simply the result of sexual intercourse between a man and woman, this world is born without any soul. For them it is only a combination of matter that has produced the living entities and there is no question of existence of the soul'

'They use science not to study nature, but to glorify atheism. Their self view determines their view of the world and their actions reflect their thoughts'. Chapter 16 of the Bhagavad Gita classifies this variety of human beings into **asuras** (having rajasic predominance) and **rakshasa** (having tamasic predominance). However certain characteristics are common. Both display **dambha**: show off what they have or pretend they have, they have **abhimaan**: pride/arrogance of the wealth status or learning they possess. Greed, lust and anger are their hallmarks. They are filled with fear and tears, though they say 'cheers '. Without the stabilising shelter of scriptural knowledge, their actions are propelled by desire. Desires become their masters. They ignore the bad in themselves and the good in others and find the need to push others down. They boast of their actions and can cause ruin and death to those around them. They flaunt their affluence and status, but sometimes the anxiety and anger they suffer cannot be hidden. Worry is also a characteristic of this class of human beings: when you do not do **Chintan** (remembrance of God's name) you have **chintah** (worry).

Prabhupada says 'The person who does not listen to the scriptures is compared to the snake that has only blind holes for ears and the one who will not say the Name is likened to the frog who has a big tongue, but can only produce harsh sounds'. The other way to differentiate the person with sattvic qualities from the person without is the concept of the 6 robbers of the mind. If one's mind and intellect have been stolen by these guys, he/she is surely heading towards spiritual bankruptcy. Keep them in check, your bank balance is safe.

1. **Kama:** lust, desire that arises from the senses, desire without boundaries, desire that overpowers you. Not all desires are bad. Kama is the desire that makes you weaker.
2. **Krodh:** anger, when my desire is not fulfilled, I get angry. When I am unable to control my anger, there is a lot of collateral damage.
3. **Lobh:** greed. While contemplating the objects of the senses, attachment develops, when my desire is fulfilled, I get greedy for more.
4. **Ahankar:** sense of false ego, pride: I have achieved so much, I possess so much, my children are so smart. I get attached to all that I have, worry that I will lose it, and spend a lot of effort protecting what I consider me and mine.
5. **Moh:** Delusion. When there is delusion, what is right appears to be wrong and what is wrong appears to be right. The means of knowledge is faulty, therefore, the understanding is faulty. The person who has delusion jumps to wrong conclusions, because his concepts are distorted.
6. **Madsaria:** jealousy.

Two of the 6 robbers, lust (**Kama**) anger (**Krodh**) require special attention:

Kama The psychology of **Kama** (overpowering desire, desire that is without boundaries) can be understood better when one understands the Vedic definition of mind and its relation to the senses and body.

Mind: Vedic tradition considers the mind an instrument (**antarkarna**) which has four components:

1. **Citta:** imprint of memories from the present and past lives that shape our likes and dislikes. It can be compared to pebbles thrown into a lake which collect at the bottom. We may not be aware of these impressions (**samskaras**), but they color the glasses through which we see the world.
2. **Manas:** The receptive component of the mind that deals with sensory input. Information keeps flowing in. Our manas can be a well sorted out filing cabinet or an unorganized heap of mental stuff.
3. **Buddhi:** the intellect. Intellect needs to be trained and developed to have discrimination and make decisions. It is the seat of cognition and conition (will power).
4. **Ahamkara:** the sense of identity or ego that one experiences.

So, Kama can reside in the 5 senses (vision, touch, taste, smell and hearing), or in the manas (receptive component of mind) or in the intellect (buddhi) The senses are different outlets of kama. Lust is reserved within the body but given vent through the senses. All sense organs are the external outlets of the mind. Mind understands the language of the senses. The senses themselves cannot function without the mind. Mind reacts to the stimuli of the senses, emotion, love, anger are expressed as thoughts. The mind does not have power to decide. The intellect has the power to decide. The senses perceive what they like and dislike, the receptive component of the mind (manas) either loves or hates it, the intellect then tries to justify the choice. When the desire comes to reside in the intellect, it becomes very difficult to remove. In the Bhagavad Gita, examples are used to explain: When kama resides in the senses it is compared to fire and smoke (we can see the fire through the smoke). When Kama resides in the manas it is compared to dust covering the mirror (takes more work to be rid of) but the kama in the intellect is like the helpless embryo in the womb (needs 9-month perseverance period). This is because kama in the senses covers knowledge, but in intellect destroys knowledge. In the Bhagavad Gita (2:60) we read 'the senses are so strong and impetuous O Arjuna, they forcibly can carry away the mind even of a person of discrimination who is endeavouring to control them'. The book elaborates (2:67) 'As a strong wind sweeps away a boat on the water, even one of the roaming senses on which the mind focuses can carry away a man's intelligence.'

Kama is a voracious eater, who wants more and more. The more you fuel a desire, the stronger hold it has on you. if he is not satisfied, he brings in Krodh (anger). Failure to integrate sense, mind and intellect is the cause of failure to overcome Kama. Intellect knows the act is wrong, tries to tell the mind, the mind does not listen gives in to pleasure. repeats pleasure seeking behaviour, pleasure seeking tendency (**vaasna**) is strengthened. Neurons that fire together wire together. You drink coffee for 3 days, on the fourth day your coffee vaasna is building. Pleasure seeking tendencies (**vaasnas**) are ruts in your mind. Fulfilling the same desire again and again leads to formation of a bad habit: the ruts become deeper and deeper: Then you follow the Law of Momentum: the more you do it, the harder it is to stop. When the stone is rolling downhill, it easily moves in a straight line but to turn it needs more energy. You need more energy, will power to get out of the downward spiral and break the habit.

So how do we overcome kama? How do we deal with these destructive desires and habits? To destroy an enemy, we need to locate him, go into enemy territory. So, to illustrate, I want that beautiful watch in the store/online display. My eyes see it, before they can get captivated, I close them, move on or turn the page. I have stopped the invasion. We can cultivate control over a desire, by looking at it objectively as soon as it arises within us. If you do not nip the desire in the bud, it will overpower you. When the milk in the pot gets hot, bubbles start arising. As the heat increases, the bubbles increase and rise higher. if you do not switch off the stove in time, the milk will overflow. Look at the desire, is it good or bad for me? I am diabetic, I like ice cream, but it is bad for me, so I replace the sweet desire with another desire. A desire needs a hook, you hook it, look at it and give in to it, but if you ignore it and do not look at it, it will go away. If the senses are regulated by the intellect, it is easier to overcome kama. Mind is more restless therefore better to deal with intellect as long as one does not justify with faulty logic. Kama can only be overcome by rising above it, by remaining at a level of senses and mind we cannot destroy kama. Intellect is transcended by meditation.

if one engages the intellect and mind through consciousness into the higher ideal, even though the senses are very strong like serpents, they will become serpents with broken fangs.

Krodh If this guy loots you (you are unable to keep your anger in check), you are in serious trouble. There are two main varieties of anger:

1. **Implosive:** Anger is suppressed (lava inside). Long term harbouring of anger within yourself is like keeping a

stranger in your house without rent. Tara works full time and looks after her family and home. Constant fatigue and pain were plaguing her. I talked to her, trying to put a finger on the root cause, it was neither the hip joint nor the anemia. There was a simmering grudge at having to do too much all the time without appreciation or reward. The unspoken anger transmuted into pain.

2. **Explosive:** Anger is expressed (lava outside). Sheena was 6 months pregnant with her second child, when upset with the many quarreling extended family members that she had to put up with, ravaged with financial problems, she chose an inopportune moment to have an argument on the driveway with her husband. Tempers flared, she hit the windshield of her own car with the available cricket bat. Not only did the windshield splinter, but the police appeared because a nosy neighbour wanted to play good Samaritan. She was ordered to stay away from her husband and spent the next three months of her pregnancy, homeless and pleading with the law. A big price to pay for one moment of indiscretion.

Another one of my patients, Paul (name changed) paid a similar penalty for his inability to control his anger. He was shouting at his mother for some reason, in front of his six-year-old son. His wife intervened, saying the child should not be witness to such behavior. Those few words provoked him to turn his anger on to her, hitting her and giving her a black eye and other injuries. His wife moved out with the children. He spent the next three days in jail.

Why this extreme damage? Because anger suppresses intelligence. Anger is one letter short of danger. It is like holding a piece of burning charcoal in your hand and wanting to throw it at the person who angers you. Your hand gets burnt first.

Three types of people are more prone to anger, but none of us is invulnerable to this emotion:

1. Control freak: when one loses control over others or thinks one has, he/she gets angry.
2. Perfectionist: angry when everything is not 10 out of 10.
3. Enjoyment maniac: In Hindi it is said maaza, maaza, saaza, saaza (fun, fun-punishment, punishment). When someone/something thwarts my fun, I get furious.

When I counsel my patients on anger management, I give the following suggestions.

When you are angry:

Disassociate yourself from anger. I am not angry; my mind is angry. We make halwa by keeping the **kadai** (cooking vessel) at a safe distance. In India and some middle eastern countries, Halwa is a type of sweet that is made by continuously stirring the concoction while it heats on the stove. But we do not burn ourselves, even while making it because we are away from the hot vessel (kadai) and its contents. Also, the regulator of the stove should be in your control. If you cannot keep your anger level in check, the halwa will get burnt.

When angry, do not speak,

When the other person is angry:

Do not get angry at the person who is angry. If it is a person who matters to you, like a spouse- listen, listen, listen. Relationships between couples deteriorate when couples do not listen to each other.

Do not tell the angry person not to get angry, mirror his anger nor tell him to shut up. He is like champagne spouting out when the cork is released-He cannot stop the words rushing out.

As in the famous story of **Shiva** goes, drinking up the poison from the ocean, do not spit out your anger (express it), nor swallow it (suppress it). Hold it in your throat and dispose of it at the correct time and place. That is why Shiva's throat is blue. Yes, it is true. Anger is a powerful emotion, use it wisely. You may not actually be angry but you can use anger as a strategy to improve the lives of persons you care for, like a father using a show of anger to discipline his growing child.

CHAPTER 9
THE LAW OF KARMA

When I question different people across the age spectrum about religion and God, I get varying responses. I asked my teenager grandson – he said religion and God are important but he will rather talk about tennis, school and friends. His father, who is mostly preoccupied with his role as father, says he prays to God regularly to keep him and his family safe. He devotes perhaps 2 to 5 minutes of the entire day to the subject. My 93-year-old mother, a devout Muslim all her life, dedicates about 2 hours to reciting prayers. These are in Arabic; she does not understand the language, but the recitation gives her a good feeling amidst the desolation of her lonely day.

Her theistic faith, like yours Jacob, propounds certain do and don'ts. Perhaps, it was the correct way to teach during those time periods when these religions were started, but if one understands why one does something, it becomes easier to remember and practice.

When I was doing my family medicine residency in Canada, at the mature age of 48, I had a few mental cobwebs, the younger physicians did not. So, I struggled with the seven steps required to be done to insert a urinary catheter. But once I understood why one does which step, I succeeded.

In a similar manner, if one pauses to understand the Vedic concept why one needs to do what one needs to do to acquire the sattvic qualities, do sattvic tapas and make the container dazzle, the steps fall in place.

However, unlike medical procedural knowledge, you cannot say "prove it" How do I know what you are stating is the truth? I will reply: "How can I ask you to see, when you do not have the eyes to see?" Swami Vivekananda asked his guru, Ramakrishna Paramhansa the question: Do you see God? To which Ramakrishna replied: 'I see him as much as I see you.' We just need those spiritual eyes. Our present equipment fails miserably.

The ordinary intellect stops short at the spiritual border. You can use a boat only to cross the river. Once the river bank is reached to go forward on your journey you need another mode of transportation. When you need to acquire transcendental knowledge, your mind and intellect has to transcend into another plane. To put it differently, we need the correct instrument, we cannot use a microscope to measure size or use litmus paper to see a virus.

Purify mind – use intellect to study the scriptures-understand the principles- assimilate- apply to your day-to-day life. When the purified mind is free of the din of noisy thoughts, the knowledge flows in easily.

What is the essential crux of this knowledge?

It is to realize that each living being from plants to human beings, a total of 840,000 species (according to Vedic texts) is a soul/spirit/Consciousness and all of these are a part of the whole – the Supreme Consciousness.

Each tiny bit of consciousness is immortal and each tiny bit is part of the whole. The Bhagavad Gita explains (2:20): For the soul, there is neither birth nor death at any time. He has not come into being, does not come into being, nor will come into being. He is unborn, eternal, ever existing and primeval. He is not slain when the body is slain.

Prabhupada describes the soul in an essay given as an address at the university of Nairobi – *Build your Nations on the spiritual platform" (from the book: The science of self realization published in 1977)* 'There are innumerable particles of spiritual atoms, which are measured as one ten – thousandth of the upper portion of a hair. Because we have no instrument to measure the dimensions of the soul, it is measured in this way. In other words, the soul is so small that it is smaller than an atom. This small particle is within you, within me, within the elephant, within gigantic animals, within all men, in the ant, in the tree, everywhere. However scientific knowledge cannot estimate the dimensions of the soul, nor can a doctor locate the soul within the body. Consequently, material scientists conclude that there is no soul, but that is not a fact. There is a soul. The presence of a soul makes the difference between a living and dead body. As soon as the soul departs from the body, the body dies. It has no value. However great a scientist or philosopher one may be, he must admit that as soon as the soul departs from the body, the body dies. It then has no value and has to be thrown away. We should try to understand that the soul is valuable, not the body. Because the soul is a part and parcel of God, it has Godly qualities. We living entities are innumerable, there is no limit to our number. God, however, is one. He is also living as we are, but we are minute particles of that living force. For example, a particle of gold is the same in quality as a gold in a gold mine. If we chemically analyze the ingredients in a small drop of (sea) water, we find all the ingredients that are to be found in the vast ocean. In a similar way we are one with God, being his part and parcel. God/Supreme Consciousness is the original root of the entire cosmic manifestation. God is the supreme will, the supreme power, the supreme independent one and we beings are part and parcel of him and have these qualities in minute quantity. In the Vedas it is stated that God is the supreme living force, among all living forces. He is also supplying the necessities of all the living entities' In another part of the same essay, Prabhupada writes: 'people who do not believe in the soul are in a most unfortunate condition. They do not know where they came from nor where they are going. Knowledge of the soul is the most important knowledge, but it is not discussed in any university. But what is the constitution of this body? What is the difference between a dead body and a living body? Why is the body living? No one is presently studying these questions.

Yet, this same knowledge has been given in the Bhagavad Gita, it is up to us to accept it. Why should we accept it? because it has been spoken by Krishna and Krishna is infallible. Actually, it is the only process by which we can understand God. To understand God by our own speculation is not possible for God is unlimited and we are limited. Our knowledge and perception are both limited, so how can we understand the unlimited? If we simply accept the version of the unlimited that God himself has given, we can come to understand Him. That understanding is our perfection.'

'Speculative knowledge of God will lead us nowhere. If a boy wants to know who his father is, the simple process is to ask his mother. The mother will then say "This is your father "This is the way of perfect knowledge. Of course, one may speculate about one's father, wondering if this is the man or that is the man and one may wander over the whole city asking "Are you, my father? Are you, my father?" The knowledge derived from such a process will always remain imperfect. One will never find his father in this way. The simple process is to take the knowledge from an authority in this case the mother. She simply says "My dear boy, here is your father" In this way our knowledge is perfect. Transcendental knowledge is similar (*From – Real Advancement means knowing God, The Science of self realization by A.C. BhaktiVedanta Srila Prabhu pada*)

The soul of the human being is unique in the sense that only when we are in the human form, we have willing, feeling, thinking and desiring and it is possible to realize the connection between us and God (Krishna/Supreme Consciousness). Other living beings, like our pet dog and cat do not have this ability. So, if we just spend our lives like they do to eating, sleeping, defending and mating, though we may use computers, build skyscrapers and drive cars we have just wasted our human potential and the chance for God realization (to realize that we are tiny part and parcels of God)

The question then is why do we continue this futile endeavour? Why do we keep watering the leaves and flowers of the plants instead of the roots?

Prabhupada points out that the plant grows, bears flowers and fruit only when the roots are watered.

He has an important point. We keep on doing the act of watering, (service) because it is our intrinsic nature to serve. Actually, we do always keep rendering service to someone or something. If we have no one to serve, sometimes we keep a pet cat or dog and render service to it. Or we may choose to serve Mammon, (trying to accumulate as much wealth as we can). But the accumulation of wealth does not lead to complete fulfilment nor does the pet dog or cat.

We try to serve because we want to connect, none of us like being lonely. We want to connect because we are not discrete entities but part of the whole. a part that has forgotten that he/she is a part of the whole. The Vedic concept of non duality reminds you – we are not two, not many, just one. if the teeth bite the tongue, we do not punish the teeth by extracting them. Both of them are you.

The hand is part of the body, but is still a hand. The hand does not grasp food to feed itself but delivers food to the mouth so that it can be processed in the stomach and intestines and in turn gets energy bundles to function well. The hand does not ask the stomach for a thank you because it knows that both are part of the same body. In a similar fashion, remembering Krishna, doing work for Krishna, through service to other living beings both human and non human, gives fulfillment to our self.

It is also the intrinsic disposition of all living beings to attempt to overcome suffering. At the animal level, it is limited to satisfying hunger and escaping predators. The human being in addition desires delicious food, a good house, car, a fat bank balance and periodic vacations to ward off sorrow/discomfort/suffering. When we have these, we are temporarily happy. If there is inflation or war, we feel sad, if it snows too heavily, we have discomfort, if we have nothing to do, we experience boredom. Our constant endeavour is to overcome pain, poverty, emotional or intellectual distress, but we do not stop to think that because we are embodied beings, there will always be a cause for sorrow. Swami Priyananda in his amazing podcast on *Transcendence of Karma* says spiritual quest begins when one starts reflecting on the cause of sorrow. In his inimitable manner, he proceeds to explain the laws of transcendence: What is the cause of sorrow and its relation with rebirth, karma and non duality.

The fact that the soul is transmigrating is explained in the Bhagavad gita (2.22): 'as a person puts on new garments, giving up old ones, similarly the soul accepts new bodies, giving up the old and useless ones. When a suit becomes old, we discard it and accept another suit. Similarly, the soul is changing dresses according to desire.

Prabhu pada says in his book *The science of self realization* 'This godly particle, the soul or living force, is transmigrating from aquatics to trees and plants and then from trees and plants to insect life, then to reptile life and then to bodies of birds and beasts.'

Darwin's theory is but a partial explanation of the transmigration of the soul. The soul is transmigrating from aquatic life to plants and trees, then to insect life, then to bird life, then animal life, then human life and within human life he moves from uncivilised human life to civilised human life. The civilised life of a human being represents the culmination of evolution. Here is a junction. From this point we can again slide down into the cyclic process of evolution or we can extricate ourselves so that we no longer spin on this eternal Ferris wheel of birth- death- birth The choice is up to us. This is indicated in the Bhagavad Gita

If you are still not convinced that rebirth is real, look up *Chaitanya Charan Das*. He has written extensively as well as made several podcasts on the scientific evidence for rebirth.

Swami Mukundananda 's podcast on past lives talks about Shantidevi whose past life has been documented in the book *Shanti Devi: I have lived before by Sture Lonnerstrand*. He also has another podcast on the science of reincarnation (see appendix 4)

Swami Sarvapriyananada goes a step further and links rebirth, law of karma and non duality in his incredible *YouTube podcast Master Sureshwara on Transcendence of Karma*. This podcast achieves the superlative goal of linking the concept of the law of karma to the removal of sorrow from our lives. Death fails miserably so do not look to death as a solution from misery. Suicide and **MAID** do not end sorrow. They only destroy the gross body but you do not die, because you are not the gross body. Your soul/spirit goes seeking a new house to live in and begin the turmoil of new birth, life and death all over again till eternity. Why this concept of multiple lives? Swami Sarvapriyananda has explained it brilliantly. I have endeavored to steal a bit of the brilliance in the summary below.

In seven steps, Master Sureshwara links the banishment of sorrow to its root cause and arrives at the deep solution.

He starts with the **law of Karma**. What is the law of karma? Most of us are familiar with the saying 'as you sow so shall you reap 'You do believe this. The law of Karma just broadens the time span to include not only this life, but an unlimited life span, because the Vedic tradition, unlike the Biblical, believes that one does not have only one life, but multiple lives. In fact, we are on a universal merry-go-round of birth -life- death-birth-life-death **(punr Janam purn maran)** from which we can only step off for a few moments of eternal time to change costumes. We keep doing this till we can rescue ourselves from this cyclical motion which goes nowhere.

The **law of Karma** states that causes have effect. Actions have consequences, so whatever we are seeing in our lives are effects that must have had causes and whatever we do in this life are causes which set into motion, certain effects in this life or other lives. The body and mind are the result of past karmas, which are accumulated from ancient births by us doing moral and immoral actions.

Why this whole business of other lives? The reason is If we see situations in this life as effects, clearly as when a child is born, it has not yet committed any action, yet some babies are assigned to poor, not rich families, to caring parents vs broken homes. In fact, within a single family, I have observed one son. who as a baby was beautiful, smiled a lot, was easy to soothe and a joy to behold whilst his younger brother, born two years later had unattractive features, screamed while a three-month-old baby, was totally irksome and a terror to babysit. Why such a gross difference? The child has just been born, has not committed any moral or immoral actions? The baby has not done any karma yet.

The materialist (one who does not believe in the existence of a soul), who regards birth as a beginning of a sentence and death as the full stop, may try blame it to genes and the chance factor, but the spiritualist who regards death as a comma, understands that these traits are clearly not due to any action in this life but have been transmitted from a past life.

We also see that for what actions we do in this life, we do not necessarily get the results in this life. This person was evil, but he was not punished enough, this person is awful, yet he is having a good time. Good people suffer.

Why do good people suffer? The story of John and Juliette (names changed)

John and Juliette were both teenagers when they met in 2001 because of a total coincidence. Both of their parents decided to attend a dinner together with a common friend. John and Juliette's eyes met. From that day onwards, penniless but goal driven, John continued to date Juliette. He worked at menial jobs and studied at community college, when other teenagers were enjoying attending full time university. He delivered pizzas instead of partying on New Year's Eve, and slept not more than three hours a night for three years to complete school and still keep the pizza store job going.

In 2004, John finally succeeded in achieving his dream of becoming an accountant and presented Juliette with a wedding ring and a home to live in. The future seemed glorious and it was.

A corporate job, two children and a beautiful suburban home followed. The penniless era was left far behind. John's business acumen prompted him to leave his 9 to 5 job and plunge into the world of entrepreneurship. His business flourished but his marriage floundered. The togetherness of the early years that he felt with Juliette was replaced by constant bitching from his partner. She was enamoured with the riches and the status she now had. Fast forward to 2024. Juliette sends a legal notice to John: all your money or else!!! John is broken. He asks himself. What have I done wrong? Where has all the love of the earlier years when we struggled together gone? All my life is wasted. In spite of the million dollars in the bank account and the beach properties, the spectre of gloom looms before him. He spends his days languishing.

Why do good people suffer?

The law of Karma explains this by including the concept of rebirth: there are no effects without causes and no causes without effects. If one refutes the concept of multiple rebirths, we are faced with an illogical equation where there are effects without causes and causes without effects. The law of Karma propounds that as an embodied being, one cannot stop performing action even for a moment, except when one is in deep sleep or meditation. This voluntary action can be either a thought, spoken word or a physical action. It can be moral or immoral. The moral action brings **puniya** (merit) the immoral action brings **pap** (demerit) as an imprint on the consciousness.

Every time we do an action, we are adding and subtracting. Also, the puniya action can give **Sukh** (happiness, comfort) and the **pap** action can bring **Dukh** (unhappiness or sorrow). We see ourselves doing good or not good things, we experience pleasure sometimes and sometimes pain.

The net karmic balance for most of us at the time of death never touches zero. So, on the death bed, one has these two luggage items to be carried over as there is no more life in the body to be able to play out the **Sukh** and **Dukh** anymore. We wait to welcome the next body. The Vedic texts actually make it very interesting: The law enforcer of Death comes and tells us 'Come on my friend, pick up your luggage, let us go and figure out when we can assign you a new house to unpack your luggage in. Till then you are our paying guest in limbo.' The *Garuda Purana* (the text that deals with what happens to the soul-body complex/causal body after death) tells that it is not a fun place to be in.

No other factual evidence exists for this, if it did, we would be studying the Law of Karma in high school along with the Laws laid down by Newton and Einstein.

Swami Vivekananda said 'This is the law of karma: Good leads to good and bad leads to bad, none escapes the law' As long as past accumulated karma is there you cannot help continuing to be an embodied being and playing out the result of that past karma. Because if you have to play, you need to be in the playground and the playground in this world is your body. Past karma means the series of bodies will not stop, so if someone decides I am going to kill myself and bring my suffering to an end, Master Sureshwara says it wont work. All your past karma is still there, the terribly bad karma of this suicide will be added to it and the next life will end up much worse.

Then how can I get rid of all these past karmas? How can I stop generating new karma? We keep generating new karma because we keep on doing actions: why do we keep on doing actions? Because we want to do things that we like and avoid things that we do not like. We want certain things: money, power, status and parking spots. We try to avoid things we hate like illness, failure and poverty. Actions are inevitable but, in our case, they are being constantly fuelled by our likes and dislikes, by our constant compulsion to keep rearranging things in this life so there it is more congenial to us. Where do these likes and dislikes come from? Likes and dislikes come because we throw a screen network on what is preferable and what is non preferable to us in this world: this gives me happiness so I like it. This dirty thing is disgusting so I abhor it. We get so engrossed in the role we play as an actor in the drama of life, we forget the entity we really are and just mould ourselves into the characters of this movie played on a huge screen. The comedy movie plays on the same screen as the horror movie does.

Objects by themselves are neutral, we choose to classify them and give them names and designations. He is my brother; she is my patient. I choose to view them differently, also they are different from me.

This is the vision of duality: me and mine are separate from the others., because we forget that the world is our playground where we are playing out our karma. Just like the people in a dream seem distinct entities but yet the whole sequence is just generated out of one's mind Swami Sarvapriyananda, quoting Master Sureshwara says this vision of duality is established on the back of non enquiry. The one who realises that he is the atma/spirit, consciousness does not throw a screen network on what is preferable, not preferable nor and gets embroiled in in the web. He becomes the witness; the sorrow of external happenings does not unhinge him. He is free of the stranglehold of likes and dislikes He only performs his **dharma** (action which is right, detailed explanation in appendix 2)

Here comes the glitch. One cannot perform dharma or even conceptualize non duality until one's mind is so to say primed to understand the concept. That is why one needs to do **Karm -Yog,**

Sadhana, Seva and Tapas that is why the Bhagavad Gita was written. Master them and you are ready to move on to Master Sureshwara's last 2 steps-

To do actions even as one sees and experiences duality, without being bound by preferences. To devote time to enquire on the reality of non duality vs duality. If things do not go the way one wants, one does not mind, one does not have a problem with the display of non duality. One stops seeking happiness from good things happening outside, one does not experience sorrow when things go wrong. Instead of depending on the fragile outside world to provide happiness, one learns to experience the bliss of the true self (atma, consciousness). The whole house of illusion crumbles like the proverbial pack of cards and we begin to view the same scenario differently. We begin to understand the nature of its impermanence.

When we stop being bound by our likes and dislikes, a strange change occurs. We remain equipoised in joy and sorrow. The suffering and challenges of others affect us though these were our own. When you reach this stage, we have a feeling of oneness towards others. We feel their pain. We do not push to do only what we like.

When we stick to **dharma**, bad karma gets exhausted. You do not create more karma. you are set free. All doubts go away, all karmas burnt up as one stops trying to get happiness from the world outside. Your search for happiness ends. Master Sureshwara concludes **Sat, Chit, Ananda** (you are existence, consciousness and bliss) is your real nature. Unhappiness is not knowing your real nature. The root cause of all suffering is not knowing yourself., or ignorance of our real nature. The deep solution is to know your real self.

Swami Sarvapriyananada compares this to the situation where one is actually a billionaire, but knows not. Not knowing, the person struggles with job searches, food banks and lives on welfare, till one day he comes to know that he has a billion dollars in the bank. His search for money ends.

Although this discourse seems to apparently not include Krishna, it actually does as Krishna can be represented as the personal form of the Supreme Consciousness vs the impersonal form when we reflect on the fact that the entire material manifestation is arising from one cause. We can give the Supreme consciousness the form of Krishna, Adonai, Allah or Waheguru or seek Him in the formless aspect.

The personal concept of the Supreme consciousness as Krishna also comes to the rescue for many people because intellectualism does not belong to all. He says just believe in Me. For those without the resources to study Master Sureshwara, He provides faith as the alternative. Devotion substitutes for non-duality.

Shobana is a 72-year-old widow whose only son is terminally ill with pancreatic cancer and presently in hospital. She suffers elder abuse at the hands of the daughter-in-law on whom she has to depend on now. I asked her about her feelings, her concerns for her future. Her answer surprised me. 'I think only of my son now. Krishna will provide for the future'. Her faith prevents her from drowning in her sorrow, although she has not consciously studied non-duality.

Interestingly there are other faiths besides Hinduism like the Jain and Sikh traditions that also believe in rebirth. What is discussed in the Gita as utilizing your mind and intellect to get the true knowledge of self is termed in Sufism and in the Sikh tradition as removing the veil. Only the veil is removed from our eyes of our mind, can we see the truth. A physician colleague who practices the Sikh faith wrote to me 'We believe that we went through millions of lives to be born human and this lifetime now is our opportunity to merge with our Creator'

The Upanishads, Puranas and other texts of Vedic literature that have fortunately been preserved over the ages for us also have the same message. Seek the real goal of life. These Vedic texts of which the Bhagavad Gita is a tiny part, show us the way how this eternal cycle of birth, death, birth can be broken, so that we do not need to continue the process of renting and leaving bodies. If it is not the human form, it could be a cow, goat or a chicken. So, choose wisely when you are still human, if you eat meat, you may end up in your next life in today's inhuman slaughterhouses.

I close this chapter and my book with the teachings of Bhakti Vinod Thakur (1838-1914) who was the guru of the guru of Bhaktivedanta Srila Prabhupada (the author of Bhagavad Gita As It Is). To quote him: 'Those who have developed attachment for material things, they are running after material things, material happiness, their desire is unlimited. Material desire means only to suffer. Such a conditioned soul just thinks 'If I will be in possession of a skyscraper, multi storey building, beautiful wife, so much material opulence or if I can discover or invent new things in the material world, then I will be happy. This is the purpose of my life" Bhakti Vinod Thakur goes on further- 'Those who are devoid of Krishna Consciousness (forgetful of Krishna), they are attached to this material world, temporary material world. Bhakti Vinod Thakur says this is a great bewilderment. He says 'Oh! What great delusion they have. Those who are atheists, material scientists try to make this **dukhalaya** (miserable platform) into a **sukhalaya** (enjoyable platform) And they are also saying yes, we are making researches. One day we will find out that there will be no death at all. You will be deathless. These material scientists and logicians are making an effort to convert this **dukhalaya** into a **sukhalaya**. But the believers know that this is a temporary residence that we have. We are staying in a motel for a night or two.

Our **dhama** (destination), our goal is Purshottama Kshetra (Lord's abode.) So, we are travellers heading towards Purshottama Kshetra. At night, when it's dark, we stop to rest in the motel and wait for the sun to rise. When the effulgent sun will come out, the darkness of the night will disappear and we will catch up our path, our road and go towards Purshottama Kshetra.

So during the stay at the motel the travellers are just thinking when will the sun come out? They never sleep there. they never snore there. They never develop any attachment to the motel because it is only a short stay. Why shall we develop attachment to such a motel? One who develops attachment to the motel is a great fool'. Bhakti Vinod Thakur says this is foolishness going on.

'The motel owner is the Supreme Lord. If He would have thought of making it pleasurable, He would have done so. But it is not his desire. He does not want it. It is his desire that the motel should not be a **sukhalaya**. So, you fools, why are you trying to make it pleasurable and enjoyable? Whatever developments you may make in this material world, it will never be perfect. You cannot get pure happiness. The more we try to make this material platform enjoyable, the tighter our material bondage. The **jiva's** (conditioned soul) Swarupa (true identity) is Krishna Dasa (one who serves Krishna). If you give this up, you will become the servant of **maya** (material bondage)'.

APPENDIX 1

BEFORE YOU START THE ACTUAL STUDY OF THE BHAGAVAD GITA

It is easier to learn when one does not know and knows that he knows not. Sometimes our own pride prevents us from seeking help. One needs to question what one is seeking in life. Maybe your answer is 'I do not know'. The Gita is the question- answer book to turn to. The structure of the Gita is first the teacher tells what he is going to tell, next he tells, but in terse verses. It contains 720 **shlokas** (verses.)

I compare it to **Toronto Notes**. Let me explain: My family and myself emigrated to Canada in the year 2000. I was then a practicing radiologist in Mumbai, India.

In 2002, after going through one of the most difficult periods of my life, I decided that, either I obtain a medical license to practice in this country or pack up my bags and return to India. I had to study medicine school syllabus all over again after a gap of 25 years. Sticking out like a sore thumb on the Canadian medical marketplace, no money, no recognised degree, no status, with the help of fellow have-nots (the international medical graduates who like me either drove taxi cabs, worked in MacDonald's or did security guard jobs), I started studying for the qualifying exams. The Bible recommended was the **Toronto Notes**. After four months and one failed exam attempt, I understood I needed other books, help, classes to understand the total sum of what was presented in the terse paragraphs and bulleted lines. The knowledge was there, but so tightly concise that I could not assimilate it. I started daily trips to the McMaster University library which was situated in another city, pored over the classical textbooks, till what was written in the Toronto Notes could be understood and then memorised.

So it is with the Gita, a superficial reading does not suffice. You need to study with the help of commentaries, study groups or classes, so that your understanding improves and knowledge increases.

Many commentaries are readily available on YouTube podcasts. My favorite swamis whose podcasts I really value are Swami Sarvapriyananda, Swami Nikhilananda, Swami Tyagananda and Chaitanya Charan Das. Online study groups are also available. Organizations like ISKCON, Chinmaya Mission and Vedanta Society are great resources.

The first step one needs to do is regular study. Devote one specific hour of your day to your study and time for sadhana because only reading is not enough. Same time, same place helps. One needs to understand the knowledge before one can apply it to one's daily life. As our self identity becomes clearer, our world view becomes less distorted.

Yes, studying the Gita and applying the knowledge given may seem a mammoth, near impossible task, but if we continue living the way we live, we will always be the way we are. As with others before us, old age too will soon loom on the horizon as a period of distress and suffering spent in isolation or in a nursing home or ended by **MAID** unless – Unless we divert and zoom into the Bhagavad Gita or a similar track now.

This book has been written in the hope that you will.

APPENDIX 2

MEANINGS OF WORDS IN BOLD AND MORE

Addiction: intention to do repeatedly, what one does not really intend to do *(from Chaitanya Charan Das)*. To get rid of an addiction, avoid the situation that fuels the addiction. Every time you submit to the addiction it becomes stronger.

Annamayakosha: the gross body, the one we can see. Allopathic medicine classifies the human structure into mind and body and the body into the different systems- digestive, cardiovascular, respiratory, excretory, nervous etc. In contrast, Vedic knowledge describes the mind and body of the human being as envelopes around the **atma** (consciousness, self). The outermost is the gross body annamayakosha which is made up of the food we consume. Kosha means envelope, anna is food. Next is Pranayama Kosha: envelope of the systems that make the gross body function: the processes of breathing, digestion and excretion, circulation of blood and lymph as well as reproduction. The envelope closest to the **atma** is the anandamayakosha Kosha, the subtle body.

Atma: consciousness, spirit, our real self

Avatar of God: God takes on a human form

Battle of Kurukshetra: The battle between two warring cousins, which is also the background where the Bhagavad Gita was spoken.

BhutyagnAsangahabuddhi: mind free of attachment

Bhava: feeling of a mix of affection, devotion and love

Danam: Charity

Dhama: restraint of senses

Dharma: Though the word Dharma can be interpreted as religion, ethics, moral code etc, it also signifies the way of righteousness and living in harmony with the rest of creation. *Gaurang Das Prabhu* gives the simplest explanation: Dharma can be interpreted as duty, but the concept of duty varies as per our identity. Am I the son or father? CEO or citizen? We need to know who we really are. Once we can understand our true identity, we can be aware of our true **dharma** and then follow it consistently.

Dhyana: focussed attention.

Dhih: purified intellect where there is decrease of desires, attraction, repulsion, ego and excessive work. During meditation, dhih increases.

Deha: body that can be burnt or will decompose

Dhata: nourisher

Dehi: embodied

Desire: How long will it keep me happy? If I do not have it, will it make a difference? Let not our prayers to Krishna, (or other personal God) be for fulfillment of desires, let Krishna be the fulfillment of desire. *Borrowed from Chaitanya Charan Das.*

Dhih yon a prachodaya: let our intellect be awakened so that all of us have a vision of our real selves. This is the last line of the powerful Gayatri Mantra.

Garbo Upanishad: The Upanishad that describes the development of the fetus in the woman's body.

Garuda Purana: The Vedic text that describes the journey of the soul after the death of the physical body.

Hatha Yog: A discipline that deals with practices to improve flexibility and overall health of the body.

Japa: chanting of holy names by oneself in solitude

Jnanam: knowledge

Jneyam: object of knowledge

Joy: Anything that gives me joy in life can be taken away from me if the source of joy is outside me. If the source of joy is myself alone, it will remain constant and never leave me.

Karma: impression created on the consciousness by whatever action (thought speech or physical action) that we perform.

Kirtan: chanting or singing of holy names and songs as a group

Ksetra: field

Ksetra-jnam: knowledge of the field

Krishna Consciousness: How do I personally interpret the term Krishna consciousness'? For me, it means living one's life conscious of the presence of the Supreme Consciousness. Though the goal of self realization (knowing you are the atma/soul, not the body and mind) may seem miles away you inch toward it slowly each day.

Lie: one tells a lie for two reasons, either one wants something or one is scared of something.

Mahabharata war: war between warring cousins in which Krishna plays a pivotal role (see also Battle of Kurukshetra)

MAID: Medical assistance in dying. allowed for persons with a reasonably foreseeable death. In 2022, there were 13,241 medically assisted deaths in Canada. MAID tourism happens in Switzerland. In the Netherlands, the Assisted Suicide Act has been in effect since 2004 (source Medical Post magazine. January 2024 issue)

Meditation: is a state not a process. Mindfulness is not meditation. There is also a difference between meditation and concentration. Focussing on breath is a good initial practice. If you want to find yourself, you need to focus on the self. The sun does not burn because sunlight is dissipated, however, by focussing the sunlight on a lens, we can burn paper. Focussing the mind by concentration on a single point for example the breath quiets the mind.

Naishkarmya siddhi (Realization of the absolute) treatise on Advaita Vedanta written by Master Sureshwara

Nitya karma: obligatory duties:

Duty to body: give good food, keep clean, adequate sleep and exercise.

Duty to mind: feed it love and compassion, so it does not go begging outside

Duty to intellect: discipline it, so that it can discriminate between what is good **(Shreyas)** and what is pleasant **(Preyas)**

Duty to family: keep family united, maintain harmony

Duty to country: we get benefits from our country, so we need to give it our due.

Duty to society: give back to society, take care of animals.

Duty to environment: we get water, free air do not pollute the environment

Positive thinking: this is not from the Gita but from a person who believed in the Gita (*K K Med Talks on positive thinking*) Dr. Kishen Aggarwal would say if you have negative thoughts, you can change it in 3 different ways: think opposite, think positive, think different. Substitute negative words for positive words. Remove three letter words like bad and mad from your vocabulary. Ask yourself, what I think will help me, will it help others? Do not compare yourself with others.

Prasad: food that is offered to God and the deities

PurushArtha: Aim of life of human being

Preyas: a temporary solution to a permanent itch

Purush one who pervades the purv (city) of the body

Pralabhad karma: old impressions (from past and present life) that have already started manifesting. This is different from Sanchita karma where the results have still to unfold (still in the bag)

Pranayama: The translation of the word **pran** is life, **Vayu** means air and **yama** means practice. It is the practice of breath control which is effective for quieting the mind. One cannot focus on the breath and think at the same time.

Punr Janam purnr maran: recurrent cycles of birth and death

Reading: There is no harm in reading many books, as long we have our personal convictions. If not, we will end up confused. Keep your mind open, but not so open that your brains fall out. Depending on the source of literature, information can either have an unrestricted entry or need to be screened. As the Buddha says when it rains, do not cover the garden with silk because the plants will not get water. But the rain is acid rain, one should surely cover the garden. If we allow misleading ideas to enter our brain, it goes into the basement (subconscious level) and will be more difficult to get rid of than junk entering a home.

Self realization: realizing that one is not mind, not body but Consciousness and that is a tiny part of the Supreme Consciousness. It is also translated as realization of one's eternal relationship with Krishna and one's constitutional position as the Eternal servitor of the Lord

Sanskruti: culture, development: we cannot change basic nature but we can improve.

Sat chit anand: Our essential nature is truth, consciousness and bliss

Shlok: verse

Swadharma: role in life tailored to the individual, the Swadharma of fish is to swim, the Swadharma of a bird is to fly. It is better to perform one's own Swadharma imperfectly than attempt to do another's perfectly

Saumya Tvam: mind without duplicity

Seva: service

Sharanagati: surrender

Sankhya: type of knowledge that which describes different topics in detail

Sthitadhi: one who has steady wisdom

Stithaprayga: stabilised in wisdom

Shama: training the mind

Samadhana concentration

Samatvam: mind that has equanimity

Smile: practice the Mona Lisa smile. If you find yourself getting irritated, force yourself to smile. Even a beautiful face looks ugly, when angry.

Time Management. one needs to be aware of time stealers:

a. The robber steals your time without your knowledge for example, when you perform tasks absentmindedly.
b. The looter deceives you – time spent in scrolling through social media.
c. The dacoit takes you by force – avoidable emergencies.

Save time by avoiding unplanned activities, avoid allowing others to interrupt your work and saying no to distractions. Bad habits are also a great time waster. One cigarette costs 7 minutes. Planning ahead is a great time saver, if you fail to plan, you plan to fail. Use the 3P formula: Plan, prioritise and perform. There is even a Parkinson's law for time management: work expands to fill time, just like water fills the bottom of a basin.

Group similar tasks together to save time: If you have to do grocery, bank work and get your hair done, you get it done in one trip not three.

If you have to do routine tasks which have to be repeatedly performed, save time by doing them in the same sequential manner every time: the morning routine if performed in the same sequence everyday takes less time.

If there is a deadline for work to be completed, do not leave the work to be completed at the last minute/hour/day.

Transcendental: that which transcends, goes beyond

Upasna: put above, devotion To God

Upanishads: Vedic literature, a storehouse of ancient wisdom

Vikruti: perversion

Vikarma: prohibited actions

Waheguru: In the Sikh tradition, God is addressed as Waheguru. There is a very beautiful prayer in the Sikh prayer book. It states simply that one cries out to God (**Wahe guru**) when one is sad, but for the person who remembers Waheguru every day, misery does not touch him.

Yog: join

Yagna: noble act offered with a sense of sanctity to God, free of selfish motive and with a sense of renunciation from its result.

Yoni: body, life form that a soul gets embodied in, could be human, animal, bird or plant life.

APPENDIX 3
BOOKS I WISH TO RECOMMEND

Demystifying Reincarnation by Chaitanya Charan Das

Victor Frankel: Man's search for meaning by Dr. Michael Sabom

Shantidevi devi: I have lived before by Sture Lonnerstrand

More than a life, Sadhguru by Arundhathi Subramaniam

Death: The inside story by Sadhguru

Living with the Himalayan Masters by Swami Rama

Biography of Ramkrishna by Swami Shraddhananda

The science of self realization (published in 1977) by Bhaktivedanta Prabhupada.

Relief of tension, Depression and anxiety through spiritual living by Swami Tathagatananda, Advaita Ashram- 2008

Mind according to Vedanta by Swami Satprakashananda. Sri Ramakrishna Math Printing press 1994

Practical Vedanta by Swami Vivekananda. Advaita ashram 1995

The Gospel of Sri Ramakrishna. Sri Ramakrishna Math Printing press 1996

Selection of the complete works of Swami Vivekananda Advaita ashrama 2017

Meditation by Monks of the Ramakrishna Order. e- Gangotri Internet archive

Bhagavad Gita: Adhunik Vyakaran (in Hindi) by Ashutosh Bhardwaj

APPENDIX 4
YOUTUBE PODCASTS

TRS (The Ranveer Show) 70 Swami Mukundananda explains Secrets of Bhagavad gita, death and salvation.

TRS (The Ranveer Show) 347 Keshava swami on the 5 am club, karma and spirituality.

TRS (The Ranveer Show) 363. Dr. Pal on Gut health, the Mind-Food connection and weight loss.

TRS (The Ranveer Show) 318 Gaurang das Prabhu. Importance of Guru: Heal and grow faster.

Swami Sarvapriyananda The Princess of Kashi: – Vedanta Society of NY

Swami Sarvapriyananda Master Sureshwara on Transcendence of Karma. – Vedanta Society of NY

Dr Sundeep Ruder- Spiritual Doctors for Holistic Health Practical Vedanta/Ancient Wisdom, Modern times

NYC Vedanta The Three Gunas and story of the 3 robbers:

Swami Mukundananda: Real proof you had a past life

Swami Mukundananda: The science of reincarnation

ABOUT THE AUTHOR

Dr. Nafisa Aptekar was born in Mumbai, India, and lived there during the earlier part of her life. In Mumbai, she practiced as a radiologist. However, life took a sharp turn when the family emigrated to Canada in 2000, and Dr. Aptekar had to undergo the arduous process of obtaining a Canadian medical license. In 2007, she qualified to work as a family physician and has been practicing in Brampton, Ontario, since then. She lives there with her husband Jacob.

www.ingramcontent.com/pod-product-compliance
Lightning Source LLC
LaVergne TN
LVHW091603060526
838200LV00036B/969